Praise

"Reduced strength can have catastrophic consequences in loss of mobility, falls and fractures, and eventual withdrawal from an active life. Interventions to improve strength, such as described in *Choosing the StrongPath*, are critically important."

—Jack M. Guralnik, MD, PhD,
Professor of Epidemiology and Public Health,
University of Maryland School of Medicine

"*Choosing the StrongPath* offers a bright ray of hope to a generation known for living on their own terms: that they can truly enjoy, survive, and thrive in their golden years."

—Bert R. Mandelbaum, surgeon, author, motivational speaker, Kerlan Jobe Institute at Cedars Sinai, FIFA IOC Medical Officer for the 2016 Summer Olympic Games

"*Choosing the StrongPath* shares invaluable advice: You don't have to accept the "inevitable" effects of aging. If you want to stay in control of your health and your lifestyle for many years to come, you need this book."

—Jason Pullara, Director of Sports Performance,
Northwestern University

CHOOSING THE
StrongPath

*REVERSING THE DOWNWARD
SPIRAL OF AGING*

CHOOSING THE StrongPath

FRED BARTLIT AND STEVEN DROULLARD

WITH DR. MARNI BOPPART

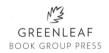

GREENLEAF
BOOK GROUP PRESS

Published by Greenleaf Book Group Press
Austin, Texas
www.gbgpress.com

Distributed by Greenleaf Book Group

For ordering information or special discounts for bulk purchases, please contact Greenleaf Book Group at PO Box 91869, Austin, TX 78709, 512.891.6100.

Design and composition by Greenleaf Book Group and Kim Lance
Cover design by Greenleaf Book Group and Kim Lance
Interior illustrations by Hard Facts LLC and Steve Stankiewicz
For permission to reproduce copyrighted material, grateful acknowledgment is made to the following sources:
From "Why I Want to Die at 75" by Ezekiel J. Emanuel from *The Atlantic*, October 2014. Copyright © 2014. Reproduced by permission of The Atlantic.
From "Military physical training: It's a problem bigger than obesity, with no easy solution" by Thomas E. Ricks from *Foreign Policy*, February 18, 2015. Copyright © 2015. Reproduced by permission of Foreign Policy. All rights reserved.
From *The Lord of the Rings* by J. R. R. Tolkien, edited by Chistopher Tolkien. Copyright © 1954, 1955, 1965, 1966 by J. R. R. Tolkien. Copyright © renewed 1982, 1983 by Christopher R. Tolkien, Michael H. R. Tolkien, John F. R. Tolkien, and Priscilla M. A. R. Tolkien. Reproduced by permission of Houghton Mifflin Harcourt Publishers Company. All rights reserved.
From "Life as the Ninth Inning Nears" by Fay Vincent from the *Wall Street Journal*, February 24, 2016. Copyright © 2016. Reproduced by permission of the *Wall Street Journal.*

Cataloging-in-Publication data is available.

Print ISBN: 978-1-62634-476-1

eBook ISBN: 978-1-62634-477-8

Part of the Tree Neutral® program, which offsets the number of trees consumed in the production and printing of this book by taking proactive steps, such as planting trees in direct proportion to the number of trees used: www.treeneutral.com

TreeNeutral

Printed in the United States of America on acid-free paper

17 18 19 20 21 22   10 9 8 7 6 5 4 3 2 1

First Edition

We dedicate this book to Roger A. Fielding, PhD

Director of the Nutrition, Exercise Physiology, and Sarcopenia
Laboratory at the Jean Mayer USDA Human Nutrition Research
Center on Aging, Tufts University, Boston, Massachusetts

In his early 60s, Fred began to wonder if there was any scientific basis supporting beliefs he had developed in contrasting his life experience with those of his friends and colleagues in dealing with the issues of frailty in aging. He began searching medical-research resources for peer-reviewed science explaining his long-term personal experience with strength training. In 1995, Fred struck gold. He remembers first setting eyes on a literature study by Dr. Fielding titled "Effects of Exercise Training in the Elderly: Impact of Progressive-Resistance Training on Skeletal Muscle and Whole-Body Protein Metabolism," presented at the winter meeting of the Nutrition Society, held at the Royal Society of Medicine on February 17, 1995.

Fred's wife recalls him excitedly telling her, "Jana, I am not crazy. You don't have to get old and weak. I was right. Exercise can save us all!" And he told her of a new medical concept he had never heard of: sarcopenia.

Amazingly, Dr. Fielding's 1995 paper described in detail things Fred had been observing as a matter of experience for 15 years. Generally, from age 20 on, there is a slow, progressive loss of lean tissue. At age 65, the decline becomes rapid and then "precipitous." The new term for this decline, sarcopenia, was coined in 1988 and was appearing in studies by the early 1990s. This loss of strength and lean mass dramatically impairs health, enjoyment of life, and happiness as people age. Physical disability becomes "prevalent" in a large segment of those over 55. Yet this decline may not be inevitable but, rather, related to a lack of activity. Older healthy individuals involved in strength training of appropriate intensity had gains in strength and muscle size comparable with young individuals.

Other scientists were working along the same lines, but it was this seminal study by Dr. Fielding that brought everything together. Dr. Fielding's work convinced Fred that he was on to life-changing science that could give billions around the world far, far better lives. Fred determined that the pursuit of this possibility would become his project of a lifetime.

When this book was conceived, Fred and Steven travelled to Tufts University and met with Dr. Fielding in his laboratory. Medicine was reaching a crossroads. Steven could see that disease born of unhealthy behavior was rising dramatically worldwide and that Dr. Fielding's overarching vision of integrating behavior modification in accord with the growing science of exercise physiology and nutrition was critical to medicine and human health in the long term, just as Fred had suspected. Dr. Fielding's vision proved a reliable map for an opening scientific frontier in health care. His guidance has been critical in the creation of this book.

"The old that is strong does not wither."

—J. R. R. TOLKEIN

Contents

Foreword

EARLY IN MY academic career, I was struck by the lack of importance given to the skeletal muscle system. This is the tissue in our bodies that is responsible for allowing us to get around, interact, play sports, burn calories, and in most cases lead productive working lives. Yet its study has typically been relegated to a single chapter in the physiology textbooks, where the fine points of muscle contraction, fatigue, and energetics are highlighted in great detail. It was not until I met my future mentor, Dr. William J. Evans, and initiated my studies in exercise physiology and metabolism that I began to understand the critically important and dynamic nature of this highly plastic and adaptable tissue. It was then that I began the long journey to understanding the central role that skeletal muscle plays in our own health and in our risk of disease.

My early work helped me understand that physical activity and structured exercise could cause remarkable adaptations in muscle that could increase endurance, delay physical fatigue, and increase strength and power. At the time, these attributes were understood to be important components of physical fitness and performance in sports.

However, my mentor drew my attention to the implications of

skeletal muscle performance and capacity, which have even greater biomedical and societal implications. Thirty years ago, we began to realize that the observed age-related declines in skeletal muscle mass and function (which we later termed sarcopenia) had dramatic and direct effects on individuals' ability to negotiate within their own environments and maintain their independence as they age. What was even more important was that we began to understand that exercise training—particularly strength or resistance training—could help preserve muscle strength and mass even in very old, frail individuals.

Since that time, through our research and the work of many other scientists, including some of my own former students and postdoctoral associates (Drs. Marni Boppart, Nathan LeBrasseur, Katsuhiko Funai, Kieran Reid, Lee Margolis, Donato Rivas, and Mike Lustgarten), we have begun to further understand the adaptive capacity and metabolic functions of skeletal muscle and the molecular basis for many of the age-related changes people experience. Through the work of many collaborators, we now understand that a regular program of structured physical activity can prevent the onset of major mobility disability in older adults. Yet surprisingly, even today, most older people and many physicians don't know much if anything about sarcopenia or about how a regular program of exercise addresses the condition.

I first met the authors of this fine book, Fred Bartlit and Steven Droullard, when they contacted me about their interest in my work on sarcopenia in 2014. They asked me if they could come visit my laboratory in Boston and share with me their thoughts about sarcopenia and their plans for this book. Somewhat skeptically, I agreed to meet with them and was at first struck by their passion for the role of exercise in the treatment of sarcopenia, their own personal stories of how they found out about this debilitating condition, and how they used exercise—primarily resistance training—to transform their own health and physical functioning.

Fred Bartlit, esteemed attorney, is perhaps the most robust and active 80-year-old I have ever met. Any doubts about Fred's commitment to fitness or training were quickly removed when I had the opportunity to go downhill skiing with him for 3 days in Vail, Colorado, in 2016. Fred is an excellent skier, and I was totally amazed at the terrain we were able to cover in those 3 perfect days.

Steven Droullard—an expert in mindfulness training, behavior modification, and attention mechanics—survived cancer and multiple surgeries, including coronary bypass surgery, only to recover his strength, function, and fitness through exercise. Steven brings to this work a strong background in mindfulness training to help overcome the biggest barrier to changing our lifelong exercise habits by making exercise a part of ingrained behavior.

I urge you to heed the advice in this book and believe that you have the power to transform your behavior and increase your physical activity to reap all of the resultant benefits, including greater strength, improved endurance, and better health. I am grateful to Fred and Steven for reaching out to me and helping us in the research community to spread the word about sarcopenia and what we can do to effectively prevent and treat this latent condition.

—ROGER A. FIELDING, PhD

Senior scientist and director, Nutrition, Exercise Physiology,
and Sarcopenia Laboratory, Tufts University

A Journey to a Stronger Life

WITHOUT MUCH THOUGHT for longevity or aging, in my mid-50s a catalyst changed me forever. I was sitting in a bar, waiting to meet a friend, when I heard the door swing open. I turned my head and caught sight of the most beautiful woman I had ever seen in my life. She was lean, athletic, and, although she wore not a bit of makeup, her skin was radiant. Despite my confidence, it was clear that she wanted no part of me.

Hopeful and never one to quit, the next night I returned to the same bar around the same time. As I had hoped, she did too, and this time she spoke to me. She even accepted an invitation to dinner the following week. During that dinner, we talked for hours.

When I met Jana, the woman who would become my wife of over 30 years, I wanted to impress her. I decided a good way to accomplish this was to go to the gym with her. However, the visit did not go as I had planned. Instead, she scoffed, "This is ridiculous. You're wasting your time. This workout is not difficult enough to get results."

Jana's candor prompted me to do something I had rarely done in my life: I asked for advice. She said I had to join a "real gym" and get a "real trainer." I did as I was told. With Jana pushing me, and my trainer driving me hard, I began lifting heavier and heavier weights. And as my workout changed, my body changed with it. Over time, although I was gaining weight on the scale, friends kept asking if I was *losing* weight. As I built muscle mass, my body grew stronger and tighter.

During the 15 years that followed, I watched my dad as he aged. His muscles deteriorated and his strength waned. I saw depression overtake him as he realized that he had wasted a big chunk of his life. I vowed that I would not squander the last 30 years of my life and, instead, would make them better and better.

As my buddies began retiring and moving to assisted-living facilities, I continued to ski, swim, golf, and run. None of those my age who I have worked and played with over a long career are still competing at the hard things of life. Not one.

And now, at 85, I am much more powerful than when I was a 22-year-old US Army Ranger. I am a stronger, faster, and braver skier than I was at age 40. I am winning more at golf than ever in my long life. I am still an active trial lawyer who has the power and life force to work harder and longer than ever before in my life.

I have stuck to my wife's advice about resistance training and still do it with increasing weight to this day. As the years passed, I saw more and more how right she had been and I continued to jack up the intensity of my workouts. I began to see that I was still changing, evolving, and becoming increasingly different from my peers, both physically and mentally.

A FACT-FINDING MISSION

Filled with curiosity about the benefits of my own path to strength training, I sought out and found large medical reference databases like

Medline, which collect peer-reviewed medical research. I wanted to learn about muscle strength and its impact on my health. Much of the information was not easily understood by novices like me, but I gradually learned how to tease out the hard science. I was stunned by what I discovered. Muscle mass and strength are critical to physical and mental health, and both add to the enjoyment of life. Hundreds of studies, Nobel Prize–winning research, and fascinating angles were becoming increasingly clear and accessible to me. I couldn't soak up enough on the topic.

Medical science confirmed everything Jana had taught me years ago. She encouraged me to write a book so that I could share my findings with others. It was a noble idea, but I needed more answers first. I had anecdotal evidence based on my own experience: I was well into my 60s when my skiing buddies suddenly stopped joining me. They had tons of excuses, ranging from being too busy to having too much work. But I was still going strong, challenging myself more and more. While they were slowing down, I was taking more difficult runs. It started to sink in that they might have been getting too frail to tackle the slopes with the same vitality we'd all once shared. They may have chalked up their slowdown to the natural aging process. But I knew that my strength training had had a positive impact on my overall health, and I wanted to learn more.

At Jana's suggestion, I decided to go on an intense fact-finding mission. I focused my search on strength training and on muscle deterioration as a consequence of age. I wanted to learn all I could. Like a journalist, I started my own investigation in the same way I used to begin an important case: I sought out experts, searched periodicals, found websites, asked questions, went to conferences, and absorbed everything written on the subject. I made it my job to soak up anything I could find on aging and the notion of wasting away as the years unfolded. Mostly, I was curious if any scientific discussion existed on what we could do to prevent what most people saw as the result of the natural progression of time: frailty.

One of my first stops was my son-in-law, Ben Marcus, a brilliant surgeon at a world-famous university. His initial response under-scored what most people believed: "It's just what happens when people get older." Still, he agreed we should investigate further, and together we sought out more information, more research, and more experts. The results of our initial findings were disappointing. Most medical professionals we spoke to thought frailty was an inevitable part of the aging process.

However, we refused to accept that answer. If *I* could stay strong and vibrant, couldn't everyone? I wasn't special in any way. I simply made the time to do resistance training.

A MOVEMENT EMERGED

I didn't set out to start a movement. I simply began talking to people out of curiosity about strength and aging—basically to anyone who would listen. Along the way, I met Steven Droullard, an expert in atten-tion mechanics as they relate to my aging paradox and my quest to understand why some people remained strong and gained strength while others walked off into aging with the acceptance that with each day, they would become weaker and weaker.

Steven, though 20 years my junior, was recovering from a major health crisis at the time. He had cancer and valley fever fungal pneu-monia, and he'd faced a series of other surgeries and relapses over the previous couple of decades. At my urging, Steven also hit the gym, slowly building up his strength and improving his health. In 2012, he was rushed to the emergency room from the gym, short of breath and in distress. He was rapidly diagnosed with multiple artery blockages and sent into surgery. After open-heart surgery and 3 months of downtime, he returned to the gym and his resistance training, starting over with tiny weights. Today, after diligent resistance training, he's stronger than he's ever been.

I'd done enough research by that point to know that building strength ultimately meant the difference between life and death, especially for someone like Steven who was struggling to get better. I listened to his doctors telling him to take it easy and to move, but to do nothing more strenuous than a walk. Ignoring that advice, he now enjoys enormous boosts in energy, improvement in his health, and a complete physical transformation. In a short time, he was a convert and wanted to spread the word to show others how they could control their own health destinies, so we decided to join forces on this book.

Something else emerged, too. As we talked, Steven was able to encapsulate the psychological transformation of aging and strength that occurs on a person's journey to getting healthy or avoiding frailty. Aging and the prevention of its effects were a mental game for him, even more than a physical one.

OUR EXPERT MEDICAL TEAM

Steven and I wanted to bring maximum enjoyment to the second half of your life. So that we could spread the word, stimulate the medical community, and ease the burden on our health-care system, we consulted with a team of medical professionals to verify our findings and to share additional medical information and insights with us.

As we researched, we eventually discovered that the disease we were learning about had a name: sarcopenia. But few understood it or had even heard of it. Dr. Roger Fielding, senior scientist and director of the Nutrition, Exercise Physiology, and Sarcopenia Laboratory at Tufts University, was someone who had. He's been a leader in this field for 20 years—long before anyone else knew much about it. We sought his guidance in our journey.

Dr. Marni Boppart joined us as well. Dr. Boppart's research focuses on understanding the molecular and cellular mechanisms responsible for muscle repair and growth post-exercise. Dr. Boppart conducts her research at the Beckman Institute for Advanced Science and Technology at the University of Illinois at Urbana–Champaign.

By way of this book, Steven and I want to spark a movement that challenges the accepted model of aging. We want to make a difference in other people's lives and to show them how to age well. We're motivated by that notion. We want people to know it *can* be done. We want others to enjoy life, be exuberant, feel good, have a sense of curiosity, and experience high energy. We want others to know there is another way.

—FRED BARTLIT, VAIL, COLORADO, 2016

Introduction

YOUR HEALTH AND the health of everyone you know is in a downward spiral that, if continued, can ruin your life. This spiral is driven by the most insidious disease in the world—a condition that begins affecting each of us as early as 30 years old and steadily grows worse as we age. Shockingly, almost no one—including the medical community—knows much about it or understands that this condition has a remedy. Few are teaching the remedy. Only a handful of people are doing anything to address and stop this looming health crisis that will ultimately impact all of us.

Lacking knowledge, assuming that your downward spiral is "the inevitable result of age," will diminish and destroy your own health and happiness during the second half of your life. The good news is that we all can change its course. This disease, known as sarcopenia, can be prevented. The bad news is that not enough people are aware of this disease or how to fight it. There's a clear and straightforward solution available to everyone, and it is the only way forward. By embracing it, you can make the last half of your life the best it can be and reverse the inevitable condition of age-induced frailty.

You can make your last 20 years strong, healthy, and happy ones.

How? The answer is easier than you think and it's here in this book. Know one thing: This is not another diet or exercise book. This is a collection of information and research all in one place that you will not find anywhere else. Even your doctor may lack a full awareness of all that you'll find in these pages and the path we're suggesting you take. That path is the StrongPath™. This book is the only existing roadmap to understanding what is happening to you and reversing the spiral via a dramatic and positive life change. Follow the StrongPath, and you'll save yourself an enormous amount of struggle as you age. By doing so, you'll save yourself from the effects of sarcopenia.

THE STRONGPATH

As we reveal the science behind aging and sarcopenia, we will address the mental aspect of aging, weakness, strength, and tackling strength training—which we know to be challenging for people embarking on any fitness initiative (and even more so when facing the aging process). Staying healthy and strong while aging is a choice, one that we hope you elect as you learn how strength training can have a positive effect on your life.

When writing this book, we researched muscle deterioration and strength and talked to every expert we could track down to provide the scientific basis for our discussions. During this process, we did a comprehensive test study of our own with ordinary people as subjects from various walks of life and at various stages of fitness. We focused not on weight loss, but on strength building, which is the basis for the StrongPath. Our study involved men and women, thin and overweight, athletic and non-athletic. We made sure that our selection of people was such that everyone reading this book could relate. To help us, we tapped Cullen B. Weber, CSCS, a personal fitness and strength trainer, to work with the people living in our area. In addition, for one of our subjects in Chicago, we employed Jeremy Aniciete, CSCS, NASM, and NSCA. He's the fitness manager at the spa at the Trump International Hotel and Tower.

We set out to examine the effects of regular, true strength training. Our goal was to monitor the growth in demonstrable strength that can come from an increase in muscle hypertrophy and energy system training and from the neural activation of muscular tissues. Cullen watched for and documented muscular deficiencies and movement-pattern abnormalities, recording any improvement. He also noted the participants' ability to successfully complete activities of daily living and tracked how they improved through their rate of perceived exertion. Just so you understand Cullen's equipment, it included a standard Olympic weight-lifting bar, a Matrix brand bench press and incline bench-press racks, Life Fitness brand squat and Smith racks, and Iron Grip brand dumbbell free-weights that varied in 2½-pound increments.

Later in the book, we think you'll feel motivated as you read about not only these people's physical journeys but also their mental journeys. You'll relate to someone in this group for certain—if not to all of them in some small way—as you read about their fears and the words of wisdom they have for you. You'll also learn, when you read what we have to say about their struggles, that their minds and egos interfered with their efforts initially. Their weaknesses and insecurities ultimately increased, but it also fed their desires to get stronger.

This book is your call to action. It will give you the science, background, and information you need to change your life. It's been heavily researched and is a one-of-a-kind collection of interviews, documents, assessments, and real-life case studies that we commissioned while creating a personalized action plan for you.

Our intention is to set you on the StrongPath of life. As you read on, you'll realize that you can have a longer life, better quality of life, and a dramatic increase in the control over your health and future.

So dive in, experience success, and then spread the word—not only to your friends but also to your parents, children, and doctors. The time is now.

CHAPTER 1

Our Gift of 50 Additional Years of Life

UNTIL THE LATE 1800s, the average life expectancy around the world was between 30 and 40 years. High infant mortality rates played a large part in this low average figure.[1] Major advances in the treatment of infectious disease or chronic diseases, like cancer and heart disease, had not yet occurred. Even simple illnesses or injuries could result in death, because we did not yet have the antibiotics or medications to heal them. Today, most people are reaching their high 70s. And, because of so many medical advancements, our generation and those who follow us have the potential to live even longer. The question is *Will they live better?*

While science has given us the gift of additional years, we are at risk of spending many of those years in a state of diminished quality of life. The sad reality is that many of us will wind up in a nursing home in our later years, because we have become too frail.[2] In this chapter, we'll explore why these added years do not necessarily translate to better health and why it's critical to shift our mind-set so that we value and do not waste this gift of longevity.

AN ILLUMINATING REUNION

During the last 15 years, Fred began attending reunions with the men he had served with as a troop leader and a US Army Ranger. Back in the 1950s, they were a strong, athletic, and vibrant crowd—the pick of young American men. At the reunion 60 years later, their capacity was much diminished. Many of these guys moved slowly and with difficulty. Some avoided stairs. Many had lost height and seemed shrunken. Fred had followed their careers and accomplishments throughout the years and had been impressed. They'd met from time to time over the years, but the difference between then and their most recent meeting was downright startling. Their conversations, once focused on family and sports, turned to joint replacements, medications, bowel movements, and finding retirement homes—not to mention the discussion about the passing of many of their buddies over the years. Fred remembers standing back at one point, looking out and feeling sad. The event seemed less like a celebration and more like a winding down of it all, as if this group were saying good-bye to a once-energetic era and to their love of life.

Unlike his Army buddies, Fred was taking on new challenges in his 70s, trying to capture the same enthusiasm he'd had for sports and action in his thirties. Fred was getting stronger; his friends were growing frailer. They were all once successful, talented, vibrant leaders of industry. The difference between Fred and so many others his age was stark and growing starker each year. There was a dividing line between the strong and the weak. Time had passed, and perhaps that made their obvious aging more apparent. But Fred's energy level and lifestyle compared to theirs made it clear there was something else happening. Aging into frailty wasn't inevitable. Fred was living proof that people could age and get stronger simultaneously. But how? What separated them and those like Fred?

THE BENEFIT: LONGER LIVES

Today, we are living longer and the stakes are higher. Even though our bodies had been honed and fine-tuned by Darwin's natural selection into a perfect vehicle for life on this earth, none of these genomic changes had added even a week to our average life expectancy until recently. Starting around 1880, after millennia of stagnation,[3] our life expectancy crept up slowly. By 1950, we lived to be 68 years old on average in the United States. By that time, improvements in sanitation, penicillin, and sulfa drugs had yielded the first substantial decrease in US adult mortality.[4] In the latter part of the century, living standards continued to improve for most Americans. Decreasing smoking rates and better medical care also lowered mortality from chronic diseases.[5] Most of you reading this will live on average 40–50 years longer than your ancestors born in 1880.[6] Think about that; for 30,000 years, half or more of those born were dead 40 years later. That's almost unfathomable. Because we've been given the precious gift of time, most of us think that 39 or 40 is when life actually begins.

What Causes This Increase in Life Expectancy?

- Control of infectious diseases and better nutrition spurred a dramatic rise in our life span through the first half of the twentieth century.
- In the middle part of the twentieth century, penicillin and sulfa drugs increased the average adult life span.
- In the latter part of the twentieth century, better understanding of living standards, the impact of human behavior on health, and better medical care addressed chronic diseases like heart disease, cancer, and stroke. Cardiovascular disease, in particular, showed dramatic decreases due to better medications, surgery, and reduction in tobacco smoking.

WE HAVE A CHOICE

With the gift of more years comes trepidation about aging—mostly based on the notion that we will grow frail and age poorly. Not only that, but many corporate pensions are a thing of the past.[7] Now we must prepare to take care of ourselves financially as we age. Retirement at 65 is a high-risk proposition these days when decades ago it was the norm. Personally, Fred thinks planning on retiring at 75 is more sensible. But our minds must shift: Not only are we not planning financially for this gift of added years,[8] we're also not viewing the years as potentially healthy ones.

Fred recalls a conversation with one of his kids, who asked, "Who would want to live to be 90 years old anyway?" He answered, "Someone who is 89—especially a healthy 89." People shouldn't be afraid of aging, but they *should* be terrified to age the way most of the current generation has thus far. The ability to protect this gift of time is completely in our hands.

No one fears living. In fact, longevity is a near-universal dream. What people fear is physical degeneration, indignity, disability, and suffering. Numbers like 95 or 100 years old commonly inspire visions of decrepitude, chronic disease, and suffering. These disturb and scare everyone. Everyone wants to live long, but no one wants to suffer long. The StrongPath is rewriting what longevity looks like. It secures the whole-body improvement that extends health span and life span. It maintains vigor and strength while reducing chronic disease and suffering to a minimum throughout life.

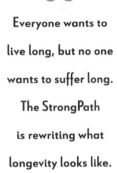

Everyone wants to live long, but no one wants to suffer long. The StrongPath is rewriting what longevity looks like.

To combat the change in life span, you need to shift your mentality: Instead of fearing age or aging, embrace it. Make it great. Few realize this opportunity exists as a choice. Being a centenarian can be a positive experience. Our behavior determines the path we choose. Here's an example: In 2015, the Huffington Post reported on a guy named Fred Winter, living in Michigan, who was 100 years old at the time and still doing 100 push-ups a day.[9] He began working on his strength and fitness around age 70. He reportedly competes (and wins!) senior games, too. So the choice is ours: We can embrace this gift of years as illustrated in Figure 1.1, or we can squander it.

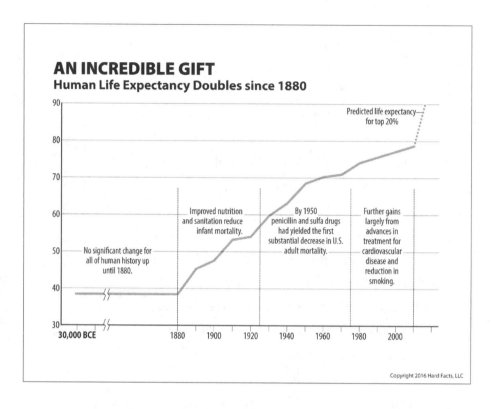

Figure 1.1. Human Life Expectancy Chart.

We are now living longer than ever before in history, nearly doubling our life span since the late nineteenth century due to extraordinary medical advances. The implications of those extra years of life are enormous. Unfortunately, many of us are not active enough, and we waste these later years because we do not realize that a change in our physical activity can dramatically improve the quality of these years. That needs to change and so does our view toward aging. We must embrace that gift by making those extra years healthy ones, not frail ones.

CHAPTER 2

A Sedentary Lifestyle: The Threat to Our Longer Life Spans

THE MATTER OF quality of life has taken on much greater significance as medical advancements have added years to our lives, making the downward spiral much longer and profound. This is a big reason we are so passionate about this cause. We're tackling it as a project, because we want to turn the ship around for this country. To our knowledge, no one—not clinicians or others—has adequately sounded the alarm on the detrimental impact of sedentary behavior on the community. If we are going to embrace the gift of longevity, it's important that we fully understand how to change our behavior, so those additional years represent a better quality of life rather than a decades-long dreary period of increasing disability, frailty, chronic disease, and mental decline.

In this chapter, we'll look at the impact of sedentary behavior on our physical bodies and learn why it is so harmful. Now that we are living longer, taking care of our strength has become critical.

THE REAL DANGER OF SEDENTARY BEHAVIOR

The impact of our sedentary lifestyle on our musculoskeletal system is pervasive: Statistics confirm that one-third of adults are inactive and another one-third is not sufficiently active to sustain health. While we lose muscle and bone as we age, we gain fat. Body fat is not only unsightly, but it also initiates a systemic inflammatory response that can harm tissue health. While some deterioration in function and health is noticeable in certain people early on, most will not be fully aware of its impact until much later in life, as the cycle of musculoskeletal tissue loss and fat infiltration progressively increase.

Two factors have created a perfect storm related to our aging population: the rapid rise in the numbers of older adults and the impact of sedentary behavior throughout their life spans. The result will be a dramatically increased rate of disabled, elderly people. Disability is a concern not only from the standpoint of loss of quality of life but also from a health-care perspective. It is unlikely that our health-care system can provide the infrastructure necessary to properly care for those who can't care for themselves.

If you don't take action now and get up and get moving by building strength, you are letting the opportunity to enjoy your personal optimal health and strength slip through your fingers. There is no "do-over." If you build your strength, you will greatly increase your health and even add years to your life. Otherwise, long before your time, you will lose your independence, physical ability, and much of your dignity. Your strength will likely deteriorate to such a degree that you'll slow way down. You may become unsteady, fall and break a hip or other bones, and become bedridden—if so, it can be a rapid decline to death. You don't have to miss the long, strong life you can have. You want to thrive. The default, a life of declining strength, is *not* inevitable; it is a needless waste of the opportunity of life that can be avoided.

That's why we're sounding the alarm bells now. Dr. Boppart assures us that the American College of Sports Medicine (ACSM), particularly the Strategic Health Initiative on Aging, has done an excellent job of gathering experts in the field to provide specific recommendations on exercise. The "Exercise Is Medicine" campaign was created to inform physicians about the importance of prescribing exercise to patients. She continued by saying that because the recommendations were not always translated or interpreted by someone with a scientific or medical background, the recommendations often went unheeded. We are committed to serving as translators, bridging the research and medical communities with anyone who will listen. We want to provide an unfiltered message about the realities of inactivity and the benefits of exercise and strength.

> If you don't take action now and get up and get moving by building strength, you are letting the opportunity to enjoy your personal optimal health and strength slip through your fingers.

OUR DREAM FOR THOSE GIFTED EXTRA YEARS

We dream of being in our 90s and doing the same level of activity—travelling the world, continuing to ski—and being those 100-year-old guys who still do their sit-ups.

To us, there is nothing more important, valuable, or wonderful than being in your 80s doing all you have ever loved and still being able to improve. You will be happier in your 80s than ever before in your entire life because you will know that you saved your own life.

WHAT KIND OF years will you have as you age? You need to ask your-self that simple question. Will they be quality years? If your lifestyle is mostly sedentary, those years will likely be unhealthy and unhappy ones. Extra time is an incredible blessing, especially if it means more of all the wonderful feelings and experiences you love and treasure. But you must take action now and get up, get moving, and build your strength—before it's too late.

SARCOPENIA: THE INSIDIOUS DISEASE

We are all prone to a disease that causes strength and muscle loss. It is called sarcopenia, and we need to understand it to combat it. For almost all aging adults, ambition is no longer on the table. Their core value has been reduced to *existing*. Everything has become all about the past; the future is no longer part of the discussion. Why? Because people aren't aging well. They are deteriorating and giving up, because they don't believe they can age better. They're living longer but not better. That's why the differences between our lives and those of our longtime buddies and peers, and our relative views of life in general, were growing more profound with every passing day. We have learned from experience that frailty does not have to come with age. In fact, it is possible to become stronger as older adults than we were in our youth.

Doubling our life expectancy means that we must focus on the quality of those extra years—with a deep sense of urgency. Sarcopenia, while still a mystery to much of the medical community, will most cer-tainly jeopardize your enjoyment of that gift of extra years, if you do nothing to combat it. The loss of strength that accompanies sarcopenia will dramatically impact your physical health. However, there is hope: You can counteract this loss of muscle tissue with strength training, which will also have a positive effect on many other chronic diseases.

SARCOPENIA IS PREVENTABLE

Let's think for a moment about how truly wonderful our lives should be today now that we have 80 to 90 years of life instead of 40. We have been handed decades of extra time to build successful businesses, be with our families, travel the world, and develop new activities and interests. Sadly, for almost all of us, these extra years we've been granted make life worse, not better. This is because everyone reading this has or will acquire a disease, a condition that deprives us of the full enjoyment of these additional years. Right now, as you read these words, you could already have sarcopenia—the insidious, almost unknown disease that threatens all you hold dear.

Beginning in our thirties, every single human being on earth develops a condition, which stealthily and steadily sucks away our strength. Every year we get weaker and weaker unless we proactively work against this default trend. The erosion of our strength accelerates in our 50s and continues to increase as we move into our 60s. There is an exponential increase in loss of lean tissue after 75.

The result is that *all* of us are trapped in a death spiral: As we lose strength, we become less active, and as we become less active, we lose more strength. Unknowingly, we spiral downward.

HOW THE SARCOPENIA DEATH SPIRAL AFFECTS OUR LIVES

The downward progression works like this: By the time we are in our 60s, we have lost a lot of our strength. This loss of strength makes it hard to recover if we lose our balance. And sooner or later, most of us suffer a bad fall—a fall that may even break a hip. The resulting couple of weeks of bed rest, or even simply inactivity, causes a further dramatic reduction in strength, which in turn further reduces our activity.

We then become much more cautious, because we can feel how close we are to falling again in our steadily weakening condition. Eventually, we endure a series of falls, each time further reducing our activity. In a few years, we can basically become disabled, confined to an easy chair, walker, or wheelchair, as the unending spiral of injury and reduced activity grinds us into worthlessness.

Please know we are not exaggerating. We have seen friends who loved life, golf, and travel become caught in the spiral until, at ages younger than 85, they died of frailty and the inability to move.

How does this happen? You know that chronic diseases are the major killers, but did you know that physical inactivity is a primary cause of most chronic diseases?[1] Inactivity is also a primary cause of sarcopenia, which is strictly correlated with physical disability and death.[2]

How can simple muscle loss cause death in so many ways? Muscles are the body's primary reserve of amino acids. They are key to the health of our immune system. When the reserve becomes depleted by 10 percent, our immune system is compromised, and we are at higher risk of infections. At minus 20 percent, we suffer from decreased wound healing, weakness, and still higher risk of infection. At minus 30 percent, we break out with bedsores, catch pneumonia, and suffer a general inability to heal. At minus 40 percent, death looms, and pneumonia overtakes many that have not already succumbed to chronic diseases.[3]

> **Muscles are the body's primary reserve of amino acids. They are key to the health of our immune system.**

We are now slowly learning that strength is critically important to enjoying the extra four or five decades we have been given. As our lives unfold, we don't think about this much. We simply assume we will get older and stay about the same in our physical strength. But it turns out that we are unknowingly facing this death spiral of lost strength that ruins our enjoyment of life long before death.

An Increase in Falls

It is useful to hear from those who are over 65 who, like most of us, always thought age was "just a number," and that their last 20–30 years would continue as always if they just "ate right and took antioxidants." The crucial takeaway here is that for almost all of us, the last 15 to 30 years of our lives bear no resemblance to what we expect. And, by far, the major reason for this end-of-life disappointment is our loss of strength with age. It is strength that is an imperative to our success and happiness as we enter the so-called "golden years."

Because of this loss of strength, one out of three people over age 65 fall every year. Falls are the leading cause of death in fatal and nonfatal injuries among older adults. Millions of those over 65 visit the emergency room every year because of falls—many of them hospitalized.

Dr. Laurence Z. Rubenstein, chairman of geriatrics at the University of Oklahoma College of Medicine (now retired), reported that 40 percent of those 65 and older fall at least once a year; 2.5 percent of those who fall are hospitalized, and only half of those live beyond another year.[4]

For those over the age of 75, the risk of being hospitalized in a long-term care facility for more than a year is high. The risk of being inactive for some period is real and pervasive. We now know that inactivity accelerates the progression of our loss of strength.

Physical and Mental Disabilities

Falls are not the only dangerous side effect of sarcopenia. People over the age of 65 have a 68 percent probability of becoming disabled in their daily activities or becoming mentally impaired. 70 percent will develop disabilities before they die, and 35 percent will enter a nursing home. In fact, many of the other common noncommunicable chronic diseases that plague the last decades of our lives are actually related to the loss of strength and can be remedied by the same techniques that cure sarcopenia. You will learn as you read on that heart disease, many forms of cancer, type 2 diabetes, Alzheimer's, and other chronic diseases may be prevented or improved when we address the causes of deteriorated strength associated with aging.

This data means that our loss-of-strength spiral inevitably ruins a large portion of the additional decades that medical science has given us. Worse, the extra years give us more time to develop disabilities and chronic diseases that absolutely prevent any real enjoyment of life.

No longer do these extra years give us more time to enjoy all the wonders life has to offer. Instead, they give most of us more time to suffer decades of mental and physical decline.

Imagine for a moment that every time you get out of a chair, walk across a room, get the mail, or pick up a prescription, it requires a lot of planning and all the physical effort you can muster. When sarcopenia has stolen your strength, it is not uncommon to think *Life just isn't worth living.*

One Nurse's Observation

In an effort to bring to life the awful experience of the downward spiral of sarcopenia, we interviewed a nurse (who asked to remain anonymous) in one of the most prestigious, high-income counties in the United States. Her report is sobering indeed: "We are seeing younger and younger patients arriving at the hospital [after a fall] in a very weakened condition without the basic strength needed to live independently."

These patients are suffering from—

- Decreased visual acuity

- Declined sensory perception

- Slowed reflexes

- Inability to cope mentally with stressful conditions

Here's what the other side of that visit looks like: When these patients return home, they're no longer able to climb stairs, so they never see their bedrooms again. They have beds moved down to the lower level of their homes and live out life in their den, office, or living room. The basement is no longer accessible. The frequency with which they leave home shrinks until it's down to never. Gone are the days of errands, grocery shopping, or even dog walking. After a bad fall, they can't even check their own mail.

Of course, then the fear of falling a second time creeps in, especially in the bathroom—where bathing becomes an issue as most can't step over the side of the tub or are too unstable to stand in a shower. Even the simple task of using the toilet becomes impossible as people suddenly can't reach their backsides to wipe.

And there's more. According to that nurse, the hygiene issues spiral: Feet and toenails can't be cut or cleaned because patients can't bend. Dental hygiene becomes an issue too, primarily because these folks can't get themselves to a dentist.

After being confined to a room at home, unable to care for one-self, hospitalization is inevitable. Once a patient enters the hospital bed with these existing limitations, his or her immediate medical issue makes matters worse:

- Many patients can't or won't get out of bed.

- Some are too weak and often too obese to even roll on their sides in bed without major assistance.

- Without the strength to move up in bed on their own, the head-board has to be elevated by pushing a button.

- Most rely on the backs of the nurses for all repositioning needs.

- Physical therapy is offered once a day, but most decline it, because they are "too tired."

These patients are also presented with constant bathroom issues. These include—

- Inability to get to the toilet without assistance

- Bedpans, which many cannot get under themselves without assistance

- Defecating in bed if they have to use the restroom and assis-tance is not immediately available

- Lying in excrement until help arrives to wash them and change the bed

- Adult diapers, excoriated and broken skin, and serious bed sores

Many patients do not have the grip strength to even open a milk or orange juice carton on their meal trays. And we are not just talking about people who are too sick to do things on their own; rather, this is how people are living day-to-day at home or in assisted-living facilities.

A Nightmare Unfolding

Let's face it. No one wants to live like this. It's a nightmare to even imagine. We all want to avoid thinking about reality as we age, but that avoidance comes at a price. Please know we're not reporting these conditions to scare you; we're simply painting a picture of the new reality, given our longer life spans.

We encourage you to visit a senior citizens' center in any metropolitan area. Notice how people over the age of 60 act and move. It will send chills down your spine as you imagine yourself or a loved one in that same situation.

The following section will share the medical conditions that drive this downward spiral. Each of us is susceptible to them. Learning about them will be useful as you understand the full scope and range of the problem.

THE SILENT EPIDEMIC THAT DOOMS US TO THE FRAIL TRAIL

We want to set the stage for the rest of this book by discussing a little more about this almost unknown medical condition that erodes, wastes, and ravages our gift of added decades of life. The disease that relegates us to the Frail Trail downhill pathway.

The key takeaway is that this is a silent, undiagnosed epidemic. We call this an epidemic, because *unless preventive action is taken*, every single person on earth, rich or poor, will suffer from the active process leading to sarcopenia.

It simply is what happens over time unless we proactively take the preventive action necessary to maintain our strength and lean mass. While our bodies' natural tendency will not change, a change in our behavior can largely prevent decline for much of our lives.[5]

As of this writing, sarcopenia is rarely diagnosed, because most medical doctors are likely unaware of the condition or how to treat it. Most of them never discuss the condition with their patients. Sarcopenia is silent, because it steadily, persistently, and without sudden symptoms can start to take away our strength and lean mass as early as our thirties.

This condition is largely a function of inactivity over time, and in modern times we have a heightened tendency to become more sedentary as we age. On average this process accelerates to take more of our strength in our 50s and 60s and increases sharply again in our 70s. As of this writing, there is no agreed upon, clearly delineated line when the process becomes a disease—sarcopenia. It is our opinion that, faced with long-term decline, we are wise not to wait to address the process of growing frailty until our lives have mostly passed and the opportunity for prevention is largely lost. Loss of strength and muscle mass can become a great threat to our ability to stay healthy and functional in the last 30 years of our lives. There are few people over 70 who are genuinely strong and active and almost none over age 80. You won't just struggle to take a walk; you'll struggle to stand on one foot and put your leg in your trousers in the morning. And from there, the final decline begins.

As you age through your 70s and into your 80s, you will find repeated little "slips," as you momentarily lose your balance. These slips can cause you to become more cautious as you move about, perhaps making you fearful to the point that you do not want to leave the house or even walk to another room in your home.

The Science of Skeletal Muscle

A pivotal factor in the ability to remain healthy and functionally independent is the capacity to preserve skeletal muscle mass and *strength*. Skeletal muscle in humans contains 50–75 percent of all proteins and is the body's primary amino acid reservoir. The functions of skeletal muscle include control of movement and posture; regulation of metabolism; storage of energy and nitrogen; acting as a primary source of amino acids for the brain and immune system; and acting as a substrate for malnutrition/starvation, injury/wound healing, and disease. Maintaining body protein mass is critical not only for remaining physically independent but also for survival. An excessive loss of body proteins results in impaired respiration and circulation due to muscle weakness, reduced immune function due to lack of nutrients, and an inadequate barrier effect of the epithelia, which likely will result in death.[6]

YOUR CALL TO ACTION

Sarcopenia is the most insidious and yet most unknown public health problem in the entire world, and it will affect 100 percent of us if we do not do something to prevent it early in life. This is a wake-up call to change your life—a call that will help you get strong and stay healthy. This isn't another vanity-based diet book or workout book focused on superficial short-term changes. Sarcopenia is real. You're not simply going to gain mobility by rebuilding the strength that's been slipping away since you were 30. You're going to regain joy of life. You're going to expand your independence. And, most important, you're going to prevent a vast range of maladies from robbing you of the healthy, vigorous life you deserve.

SADLY, FOR ALMOST all of us, these extra years we've been granted make life worse, not better, because of sarcopenia. It's a vicious cycle: As we lose strength, we become less active, and as we become less active, the rate at which we continue to lose strength constantly increases. This loss of strength makes it difficult to recover if we lose our balance, and most of us wind up suffering a bad fall. This will cause many of us to become hospitalized, which in turn decreases our life expectancy. Unfortunately, these extra years also give us more time to develop disabilities and chronic diseases that absolutely prevent any real enjoyment of life. Many of these diseases are also related to our loss of strength.

Even though sarcopenia can ultimately affect all of us, it remains widely unknown and little attention is given to its prevention. Yet it is the single greatest threat to our ability to stay healthy and functional in the last 30 years of our lives.

CHAPTER 3

The Cause of Sarcopenia

EVERYONE READING THIS book is heading down the same Frail Trail of life. To avoid this fate, what you are about to read could prove to be the most important information you will ever receive. We are confident this information will change your life in the most profound ways imaginable. How do we know this? Because learning the answers to the following questions about sarcopenia changed our lives, put us firmly on the StrongPath, and made us happier and healthier people:

- What is sarcopenia?

- When does it begin?

- How does it progress?

- What is its root cause?

- Why haven't our doctors told us about it?

- Is there a cure?

In the next few chapters, we'll answer these questions and more, so that you can fully comprehend why sarcopenia is so dangerous, how quickly it escalates, and what you can do to reverse the damage it causes. Once you better understand sarcopenia, you will be more equipped to fight it and more determined than ever to ditch the Frail Trail for the StrongPath.

WHAT IS SARCOPENIA?

The term "sarcopenia" was invented relatively recently by Irwin Rosenberg. In 1989, he first referred to loss of skeletal muscle mass and size as "sarcopenia," by combining the Greek word for "flesh" (*Sarx*) with the Greek word for "loss" (*penia*). At the time, it was thought that the degenerative process being described was led by the loss of lean muscle mass with aging. Today, it is understood that inactivity causes muscles to lose strength through a process of denervation, the loss of nerve supply that signals muscle cells to act.[1] Strength loss leads to frailty and disability over time. Loss of lean muscle mass is a trailing and serious consequence of the process. Therefore, an important indicator of the developing syndrome is loss of strength, and that is a signal for the need for intervention and rehabilitation. For example, as strength wanes, individuals tend to walk more slowly. Careful measurements of gait speed for just 4–6 meters are predictive of future disability, hospitalization, and mortality.[2]

This is all new, so terminology and definitions are still being developed. Some have proposed that "sarcopenia" should be replaced by "dynapenia," which is a somewhat more precise term for loss of strength. Just be aware that there have been several competing definitions for "sarcopenia," and we will be using the term to focus on *loss of strength*, not loss of muscle size or mass alone. This meaning was codified on October 1, 2016, when sarcopenia was recognized as an independent condition with its own International Classification of Diseases code.

Sarcopenia is now defined as loss of function in the presence of loss of muscle mass. It has been demonstrated to predict functional decline, hospitalization, and mortality in both community-dwelling older persons and residents in nursing homes.

It is now recognized that sarcopenia can be treated with resistance exercise, high whey (leucine) content balanced with essential amino acids, and vitamin D (1,000 IU a day).[3]

SINCE WE NO LONGER NEED STRENGTH TO MAKE A LIVING, WHY IS STRENGTH SO CRITICALLY IMPORTANT TODAY?

So what is the big deal about "strength"? Strong muscles evolved because they were a competitive advantage 50,000 years ago. Strength enabled killing fierce animals for food and defending our families against the bad guys.

Today, average people do not need a great deal of strength to feed their families or defend themselves. Education spares ever more from lives of hard physical labor. It is common to earn a very good living behind a desk in a comfortable, high-tech swivel chair without much exertion at all.

Most highly educated Americans value being able to avoid physical effort, delighting in things graciously being done for them. Just walking or "moving" is thought by many to be exercise enough to remain healthy.

So, again, we pose the question: What is the big deal about "strength"? Hasn't the world changed, so that strength is no longer relevant or even useful? Surprisingly, to most of us, it

> "Strength" is the reason for enjoying the extra decades of life that medical science has given us.

turns out that "strength" is the reason for enjoying the extra decades of life that medical science has given us. Strength is the missing measure of health and happiness, because there is no change in our bodies over our lifetimes that is more dramatic and dangerous to our health and well-being than a decline in our strength.[4]

It is loss of strength and physical fitness that forecasts growing risk for—

- Falls

- Functional decline

- Disabilities

- Multiple emergency visits

- Hospital stays

- Cross infections

- Nursing home admissions

- Poor quality of life

- Death[5]

On the other hand, we find that muscular strength is inversely and independently associated with death from all causes and from cancer in men, even after adjusting for cardiorespiratory fitness.[6] A recent study has also shown that in all death causes, including those that are cancer-based, mortality was lowest for men in a group representing the top third of all men in terms of strength.[7]

HUMAN MUSCLE WASTING OVER A LIFETIME

Without any other disease or injury, the condition leading to sarcopenia can cause us to lose as much as 1 percent of our strength each year after we turn 30. These changes seem subtle and symptom-free. In our 30s and 40s we just slowly notice that we are not up to doing certain things. But that's just normal. Right? And this is how the slippery slope begins.

To give you a glimpse of what can happen as we age, look at this progression of decline in muscle—starting as early as age 30—that commonly occurs if we are not proactively working to maintain our strength and fitness:

- **Ages 30–45**: What is thought of as age-related loss of strength begins around the age of 30. We tend to become more sedentary and lose 3–8 percent of our strength per decade during this time period. Growing weakness makes us feel like doing less, which makes us weaker still.

- **Age 50**: During our 50s, the rate of strength loss accelerates for most and we may experience some significant health challenges.

- **Age 65+**: As we retire, we tend to become more sedentary still and as our strength declines further, even the common daily activities of life can become challenging.[8] In 2009, 25 percent of Medicare beneficiaries that were 65 and older reported that they were having trouble performing at least one activity of daily living. Neural motor units, which contract muscles, begin to "die" or lose their ability to function.

Inactivity triggers denervation. It is important to note that muscle size is not nearly as critical as strength in evaluating the course of this disease. Strength loss is highly associated with the nervous system's inability to voluntarily activate muscles.

Accordingly, the number and magnitude of associations for low physical performance or disability are greater for low muscle strength than low muscle mass. The good news is that strength begins to return with strength training more quickly than lost muscle mass, meaning that regaining important physical abilities can occur more quickly than the time needed to significantly increase muscle mass.[9] Muscle strength is also lost faster with age than muscle mass. To be healthy long term, the habit of maintaining your strength is vital because muscle health is fundamental to whole-body health.

WHAT IS THE ROOT CAUSE OF SARCOPENIA?

Of course, the phenomenon of weakness and frailty with aging has been around for thousands of years. In fact, sarcopenia is one of the world's major public health problems. So it is surprising that peer-reviewed research only began looking into its causes in the last few decades. Accordingly, the mechanisms underlying sarcopenia are not yet fully understood. But, because discussion of remedies and cures always involves understanding causes, it is important to summarize the current state of knowledge and where research is heading.

History and Human Biology

As Theodosius Dobzhansky, one of the leading biologists of the twentieth century, said, "Nothing in biology makes sense except in the light of evolution." In this section, we will review when and how our human genome evolved and what conditions created our current genome.

Fifty thousand years ago, the world was populated with a variety of *Homo sapiens* that looked like we do now. If one of them turned up in a modern morgue, the local pathologist would notice nothing peculiar. Stephen Jay Gould observed, "There has been no biological change in

humans in 40,000 or 50,000 years. Everything we call culture and civi-
lization we've built with the same body and brain."[10]

The lesson is not that evolution stopped 50,000 years ago. Evolution
is, of course, ongoing. Rather, Gould's statement reminds us that it is
important to remember that the preponderance of evolutionary forces
that produced our species as it exists today occurred over eons. These
forces are vast in their effect in comparison to what biological change
has occurred in the relative blink of an eye during which human civi-
lization has existed. We are very much the same biological animal that
our ancestors of 50,000 years ago were. What is startlingly different
today is the environment we have constructed to live and work in that
allows for very different diets and physical behavior in the modern era.

We are just waking up to the health ramifications of this sudden
epic change in our circumstances.

Natural Selection

Our genome evolved through natural selection. Natural selection functions to select for genes that create a competitive advantage in terms of
an organism's ability to survive and reproduce. It works this way: By
chance, variations in our genetic material constantly occur, primarily
in the form of mutations. Some variations were advantageous, in the
sense that they improved our ability to survive and reproduce. Such
advantageous variations became more common as individuals with
such variations lived longer and had more progeny and thus became
incorporated in our genome.

For untold generations, genes were selected that gave early homi-
nids competitive advantages in the environment in which they lived.
Gradually, bodies changed until *Homo sapiens* became exquisitely
designed to function in low- and no-technology times like the late

Stone Age environment. And it was not just our muscles that were designed for that environment. Favorable adaptations in every part of our bodies over untold ages were selected because they created some form of competitive advantage in that environment.

Our next step, having learned that our bodies were designed for success in the environment existing in the millennia leading up to the late Stone Age, is to examine what is known about that world. This will inform us about our genes and our biology today and take us further down the path to understanding why sarcopenia saps our strength beginning in our thirties.

You will not be surprised to learn that the world our bodies were designed for was a world of intense, constant, hard physical activity: Walking and running 20–30 miles a day looking for food was common. Hunting and killing immensely powerful animals, and defending ourselves and our families, was brutal and physically demanding. Our genetic inheritance traces to the period when competition faced by all humans for survival involved very high levels of physical activity. Because there was an advantage in surviving in a harsh world of intense physical activity, variations between humans that were favorable in such a world were selected and flourished in the gene pool.

Strong, muscular humans were fitter, did better in this competitive climate, and had more progeny. Favorable genetic variations were passed on, giving subsequent generations a similar competitive advantage. This process of natural selection resulted in a population designed for and perfectly suited to survive and perform well under these conditions of intense physical activity.

We still carry the genes that allow our bodies to perform best under such conditions. And now we can envision what genome was needed to survive in such conditions. We see the images left 30,000 years ago, drawn on the walls or ceilings of different caves. At Chauvet–Pont d'Arc cave in France, we see great horned rhinoceros, buffalo, and reindeer with bone-crushing strength; gazelle-like animals possessed of great speed; and hyenas and great cats with razor-sharp teeth and claws. In a cave on Sulawesi Island in Indonesia, next to a depiction of a wild pig, we see the images of human hands that were making their way in that incredibly challenging world.

Where does this analysis take us with regard to our search for the cause of the sarcopenia-driven lifetime progressive loss of strength, which destroys much of the last 25–35 years of our lives? For the answer, we look to a new, recently emerging field of evolutionary medicine laid out by Daniel Lieberman in his sweeping book *The Story of the Human Body*. According to Lieberman, it was "extremely perilous and difficult for slow, puny, weaponless hominins to enter into the rough, tough, and hazardous business of eating other animals for dinner."[11]

To survive and procreate under such conditions, it was "essential to have the body of a professional athlete whose everyday existence required intense physical activity,"[12] suggests Lieberman.

That world is now extinct and our bodies compete in a far more sedentary world. A growing number of us earn a living by sitting with a keyboard, focused on an intellectual challenge. Our bodies were finely matched to an environment we no longer live in. Today, they are "mismatched," top to bottom, with our more sedentary world.

The Journal of Physiology published a topical review that supports the "mismatched" view. The authors observe that the survival of our late Paleolithic (50,000–10,000 BC) ancestors depended on hunting and gathering, so "the basic framework for our physiologic gene regulation was selected during an era of obligatory physical activity."[13] A sedentary lifestyle probably meant elimination. The review's authors say that in this sense, our current genome today is "maladapted, resulting in abnormal gene expression, which in turn frequently manifests itself as clinically overt disease."[14]

The "Mismatch Hypothesis" as the Possible Genesis of Sarcopenia

It was about 10,000 years ago that the intensely physical world that created our genome began to change. It was about this time that humans began to see that they could cultivate crops and raise farm animals. Early farming was physically demanding and grueling too, but a new era was dawning. A long, incremental trend toward greater mechanization and easier living increased to a gallop during the industrial age and has taken a greater leap in our high-tech age, reaching a truly incredible level today and yielding unexpected new problems.

For example, researchers followed 334,161 Europeans for 12 years. They recorded exercise levels, waistlines, and deaths. Professor of physical activity and health at the Norwegian School of Sport Sciences Ulf Ekelund told BBC News that a sedentary lifestyle is currently the greatest risk factor for an early death, regardless of weight. He added that "eliminating inactivity in Europe would cut mortality rates by nearly 7.5 percent."[15]

The number of overweight and obese individuals in the United States is growing. Of all adults that are age 20 or older, we find that more than two-thirds (68.8 percent) are now considered to be overweight or obese.[16]

And the new generation of kids in America are spending more time than ever with electronic media. Teens in the United States currently average about 9 hours of media usage daily.[17] Perhaps the best indicator of the extent of inactivity in the United States is the sad state of military recruits: "We have 18- and 19-year-old kids coming into basic training that can't skip or perform a forward roll," said Frank Palkoska, chief of the US Army's Physical Fitness Training School, in an article appearing on www.foreignpolicy.com. "They have not learned the motor patterns to execute these basic movements. It's very difficult to get a person through an obstacle course when they're starting so far behind, and ten weeks isn't enough to get them up to speed. You acquire most of your basic movement patterns by first grade, and our youth today just aren't getting the physical education time they need. Lack of fitness is a societal problem. The injury rate is developing into a taxpayer concern in terms of medical care and lost training expenses. And the lack of qualified recruits it [sic] is becoming a national security issue."[18]

Just imagine: America is full of young men whose lives have been so inactive they cannot "skip" the way we all did as kids. Regrettably, all this is more than sad—inactivity is increasingly deadly. New research in *The Lancet* suggests that inactivity is now tied to 5.3 million chronic-disease deaths annually, which is similar to the 5 million deaths tied to smoking worldwide.[19]

OUR SEDENTARY WORLD

In short, the bodies that adapted to lives of constant intense physical activity now lead totally different, sedentary lives. It is not surprising that bodies designed to operate in an intensely physical world require continuous physical activity to function as they were designed. Such bodies rapidly deteriorate when forced to function without exercise in a sedentary world.

The obvious remedy is to re-create the physically intense world for which our bodies were designed. Yet we do the opposite. When individuals are followed longitudinally over many years from early adult life, they report a progressive decline in the amount of physical activity, producing a progressive decline in strength.

Are you prepared for the medical expenses that may accompany your later years? In the next chapter, we'll take a close look at some of the costs associated with our loss of strength and decline in health to illuminate the significant financial cost of ignoring sarcopenia.

CHAPTER 4

The Enormous Cost: Life on the Frail Trail

BEFORE WE EXPLORE the cause of and cure for sarcopenia, it is important to assign a price tag to the current impact of the disease on our medical system—and our wallets. If we stay on our current course, the costs will be unsustainable, and hundreds of millions of lives will be ruined. There are tremendous costs associated with not only the urgent hospitalizations and surgeries due to falls but also the long-term care facilities that many people will require if they remain on the Frail Trail.

This isn't a fleeting issue. The costs of dealing with the frailty of aging are soaring out of control. And if our stories of the potential nightmarish death spiral ahead aren't enough to motivate you to regain your strength, then the substantial financial loss you will encounter will.

THE FINANCIAL CHALLENGES OF LONG-TERM CARE

The reality is most people will need long-term care. Only one out of four people will die before needing full-time, long-term care. The lifetime probability of becoming disabled in at least two activities of daily living or of being cognitively impaired is 68 percent for people age 65 and older.[1]

Those who become cognitively impaired or need help moving around will be barred from assisted-living facilities and will have to call on the charity of family members or pay for expensive, private home care. 66 percent will eventually be taken care of by family members. The result of family members devoting themselves to care of relatives will be a lifetime loss of more than $300,000 of income.[2]

Are you willing and able to help financially support the children or relatives who must now give up their work to care for you? All of these numbers must be considered as we assess the costs of the downward spiral on the Frail Trail:

- A study by MetLife found the actual cost of a semi-private room in a nursing home in the United States adds up to an average of $81,030 a year. For a private room, the figure goes up to $91,615. In some areas, the average can be much higher. A semi-private room in the New York metro area in 2011 ranged from $125,560 to $187,975.[3]

- The median monthly cost for assisted living in the United States is $3,500.

- The median hourly rate for homemaker services is $19.

- The median home health-care aide hourly rate is $20.

- The median day rate for adult day care centers is $65.[4]

The bottom line is essential care is expensive. Yet baby boomers are ignoring what they face. Two-thirds of them have not saved enough for even 1 year of essential care.[5] 40 percent have not saved a single penny for the care they will require. That's a crisis waiting to happen.

In a few years, most retirees will not have sufficient assets to cover basic home-care expenses or nursing home stays. Today, most of these costs are paid for by Medicare. But this coverage only lasts 100 days for a nursing facility, when people are pushed out to Medicaid. There is almost no place to go where lower-paying Medicaid is sufficient.[6]

In addition, our government has not made provisions to finance the awesome, accelerating costs of long-term care for the 76 million boomers. A commission set up by Congress in 2013 failed to come up with any solution. An avalanche of cost is careening down the mountain at us, and no state or federal agency is doing a thing to prepare us. Thus, we are facing a gigantic, looming crisis in which people need care at the most critical times of their lives, and there simply is not enough money or provisions for care available.[7]

Imagine decades of life without the care needed to make life even marginally acceptable. This is likely why a leading medical scientist has warned us "not to live too long," or, more specifically, not to live past 75, because in his view life after 75 is currently intolerable.[8]

Focus on this for a second: One of the smartest medical scientists in the United States is warning us that the last 10 years of our lives will be so awful, so miserable, so worthless, that we would be better off dead.

Remember that gift of added years of life? That makes this crisis even worse. Fred's grandfather was born when the life expectancy was 39 years. Back in his grandfather's day, frailty with aging was not much of a problem, because life was so short that people did not experience decades of life at the bottom of the downward spiral of sarcopenia. The simple, brutal fact was they died before becoming disabled.

Today, our average life expectancy is 80 years. As a result, we have 30 more years to survive with the terrible infirmities of sarcopenia. Even worse, chronic diseases have now become epidemic. As we live longer, we have more time to accumulate noninfectious chronic diseases like cancer, heart disease, Alzheimer's, asthma, and diabetes. One or more of these chronic diseases affected 133 million Americans in 2005. More than 75 cents of every health-care dollar spent nation-wide—$1.7 trillion annually—goes toward the treatment of chronic diseases. Incidences of these diseases have soared in the last 20 years. These chronic diseases have become the leading causes of death and disability in the United States and account for 70 percent of deaths in this country.[9]

THE REAL COST OF THOSE EXTRA YEARS

Medical science has learned a lot about existing chronic diseases and is now able to keep us alive with these diseases for decades. But the cost of keeping people alive for decades with these diseases is bankrupting both individuals and our health-care system. In 2010, 86 percent of health-care costs were driven by care for chronic diseases.

And it keeps getting worse. On January 22, 2009, Sen. Edward M. Kennedy stated, "The nation is facing a worsening health-care crisis that demands our immediate attention. As a nation, we spend two trillion dollars a year on care, yet 1 in 2 Americans suffer from chronic diseases that decrease quality of life and increase health costs. Estimates indicate that close to 200 million Americans alive today will have a chronic illness, and that 1 in 4 dollars will soon be spent on health care. Without basic reform, the burden and the cost of treating these chronic conditions will not be sustainable for future generations. Chronic disease can affect all Americans, and we need to focus on the steps we know will work best. The power of prevention is an essential element of health reform—the best way to address the unsustainable

> The power of prevention is an essential element of health reform.

increase in health costs related to chronic conditions is to prevent the conditions in the first place."[10]

Without prevention of frailty with aging, the costs will literally increase exponentially. From the $2 trillion noted by Senator Kennedy in 2009, "health spending in the United States grew to $3.2 trillion in 2015."[11] There simply will not be enough money in the United States to treat people.

So what are the primary approaches to prevention that might really make a big difference and turn things around? The Centers for Disease Control and Prevention (CDC) state that "four modifiable health risk behaviors—lack of physical activity, poor nutrition, tobacco use, and excessive alcohol consumption—are responsible for much of the illness, suffering, and early death related to chronic diseases."[12] The CDC says that although chronic diseases are among the most common and costly of all health problems, they are also among the most preventable and that regular physical activity is one of the most important things a person can do to stay healthy.[13]

The World Health Organization has estimated that if the major risk factors for "chronic disease were eliminated, at least 80 percent of all heart disease, stroke, and type 2 diabetes would be prevented, and more than 40 percent of cancer cases would be prevented."[14] Let this sink in a moment.

We know what is causing this growing, massive, unaffordable, debilitating, and deadly epidemic of chronic disease, which will bankrupt even the richest among nations, yet we are not seriously

> "The World Health Organization has estimated that if the major risk factors for chronic disease were eliminated, at least 80 percent of all heart disease, stroke, and type 2 diabetes would be prevented, and more than 40 percent of cancer cases would be prevented."

taking steps to do what we know must be done. The CDC tells us that the percentage of US adults 18 years of age and over who met the modest physical activity guidelines for both aerobic and muscle-strengthening physical activity in their 2015 report was a meager 20.9 percent.[15]

Approximately one-third of all US adults meet minimum levels of aerobic activity as defined by 2008 guidelines.[16] Just keeping people alive, merely lengthening lives, does not help. Indeed, this current approach ignores the critical question of quality of life. Thousands are now surging into their final decades every day. The only way to make our system sustainable is to make our longer-living individuals strong enough and healthy enough to provide for themselves and to enjoy their gift of decades of additional life.[17]

CHAPTER 5

Why Most Doctors Do Not Understand Sarcopenia—or Its Remedy

AS WE INTENSIFIED our study of sarcopenia, we conducted an interesting experiment. We began asking the wide range of people we encountered the following questions:

- Have you ever heard of sarcopenia?

- Do you think frailty with aging is inevitable?

- Do you know if there is a cure or remedy to growing frail?

The people we queried were highly educated, quite successful in business, and widely read. They all cared a great deal about their health, eating properly, and keeping informed about their health by reading articles.

You may be surprised to learn that not one of these people, over the course of 5 years, had heard about sarcopenia. Yet they all knew someone, such as their grandmother, who got frail, fell down one day, and never walked again. Without much thought, they simply expected this would be their fate and that frailty with age was inevitable.

We often suggested they ask their doctors about sarcopenia. Uniformly, they reported that their doctors mostly had never heard of sarcopenia, and if they had, it was only the most general vague recollection. None of their doctors had any advice on curing or remedying this condition. Not one.

So, the world is facing a growing epidemic of frailty. An epidemic that is degrading the quality and enjoyment of as many as 30–50 years of life. And neither the most successful, best-educated people in the world nor their doctors know much about it. Why? Well, in this chapter we'll try to enlighten you about why most doctors are missing the crucial facts and why it's essential that you educate yourself about this deadly—yet treatable—disease. The power to change your life is in your hands—not your doctor's.

> The power to change your life is in your hands.

THE STATUS OF SARCOPENIA IN THE MEDICAL COMMUNITY

As our interaction with the medical community increased, we started asking them the same questions regarding sarcopenia. Quite frequently, discussions ensued in which doctors vigorously argued that "there is no such thing" and we are "flat wrong." Fascinated with the fact that the true science concerning a serious epidemic seemed to be almost unknown to doctors, we began expanding our investigation in three areas:

- We have attended and spoken at several conferences of leading physicians in various areas of medical science. Out of two hundred or so doctors present, only three or four had even heard of sarcopenia; maybe one thought there might be a remedy for it.

- We visited senior centers where people ages 60–75 went for advice and recreation. We met with one center's board of directors. None of them had any idea what we were talking about and did not want to hear any information about it.

- We also visited a major university that had a $50 million senior wellness center, which included a wonderful gym. The medical assessment facilities capable of determining body composition, fat, and lean mass percentages were empty. A perfect facility, waiting for patients suffering from sarcopenia and desperately needing rehabilitation, was dead quiet. The medical community had not yet become fully aware of the condition.

Of course, there are some doctors around the world specializing in frailty and sarcopenia research. We attended one of their annual conferences and listened to 90 presentations. Most of them dealt with treating patients toward the end of the death spiral of inactivity and resulting weakness when patients only had few years left to save. There was almost nothing discussed on preventing the death spiral from beginning in the first place.

See for yourself: Conduct a little personal research of your own. We are sure you will find your own experience equally frightening. Just start asking friends, colleagues, acquaintances, and even your own doctors these same questions. You'll quickly see how serious the problem is.

LEADING EXPERTS DON'T AGREE

Now, if you are floored by the absence of knowledgeable medical advice on sarcopenia, its impact on each of us, and the remedies or cures that can make us a whole lot better off, hold on to your hats. It gets worse.

We were shocked when we read an article in *The Atlantic* titled "Why I Hope to Die at 75" by a leading medical expert on bioethics and aging, Dr. Ezekiel Emanuel. He is one of the most influential individuals in terms of government health policy in the United States.[1] His are the honest, underlying, rarely spoken presumptions behind the prevailing conventional wisdom on aging. He is simply giving voice to what he is sure are the hard, intractable truths that others have not had the brass or courage to articulate.

Dr. Emanuel appears to be a supremely qualified expert. He has an MS in biochemistry from Oxford and an MD and a PhD from Harvard; he completed his internship and residency in internal medicine at Boston's Beth Israel Hospital and his oncology fellowship at the Dana-Farber Cancer Institute. He has also been the recipient of dozens of honors and awards. He also is a former professor at Harvard Medical School. He was the founding chair of the Department of Bioethics at the National Institutes of Health (NIH) and held that position until August 2011, and he has made frequent TV appearances to discuss Obamacare and health-care plans.

Bioethicists like Dr. Emanuel spend their lives teaching and advising on a wide range of medical issues, including life extension, human dignity, and the sanctity of human life. So, what advice does this top scientist give us regarding living our lives with sarcopenia? Unfortunately, none. The data is factual and more than sobering. It is what aging inevitably is as long as we fail to adopt the remedy for sarcopenia.

Dr. Emanuel first describes the horrors of aging today. In his article, he states that living into our 70s "renders many of us, if not disabled, then faltering and declining, a state that may not be worse than death but is nonetheless deprived. It robs us of our creativity and ability to contribute to work, society, the world. It transforms how people experience us, relate to us, and, most important, remember us. We are no longer remembered as vibrant and engaged but as feeble, ineffectual, even pathetic."[2]

We agree with him completely that this is a fair picture of growing old for a majority today. Older years are commonly of poor quality. It is true that since 1960, increases in longevity have occurred because more people over the age of 60 are living longer. Relatively few young people die in our modern era, so even if we could save the remaining few that do, it would change overall longevity statistics only marginally. The tragedy is that older people living longer has meant more years of disability—not more healthy years.

In his article, Dr. Emanuel paints the dire picture. He notes that as people age, there is a progressive erosion of physical functioning. Dr. Emanuel's article mentions research conducted by Eileen Crimmins and a colleague, who found that between 1998 and 2006, the loss of functional mobility in the elderly increased. He says, "Americans may live longer than their parents, but they are likely to be more incapacitated. Does that sound very desirable? Not to me."[3]

In 2010, another study of the disability trends among older Americans by Crimmins and colleagues also came to the conclusion that "older Americans face increased disability" but offered an illuminating detail.[4] This study pointed to a reason for the recent increase in disability, and it was not simply longer lives. It was related to changing demographics in America's senior population and the burgeoning incidence of obesity. Obesity has risen dramatically since the 1960s, from as little as 11 percent in that era to as much as 34 percent of the American population by 2000. The changing ethnic composition of the population now reaching 60 years of age is another contributing factor. The greatest increase is occurring in black and Hispanic populations with both higher rates of obesity and lower socioeconomic status, which combine to elevate risk for functional disability.[5]

Crimmins made a simple and critical observation: "When mortality declines because people survive longer with a disease rather than because people were less likely to get a disease, there will be an expansion of disease morbidity."[6] The implication for health-care providers and policy makers should be obvious from this statement. Disease prevention is the key to better health over longer life spans. Effective prevention can also drastically lower out of control health-care costs. Powerful preventive measures are known and have been very well studied. They primarily consist of modifying unhealthy lifestyle and diet habits. More on that in a moment.

Dr. Emanuel continues by referencing mental disabilities that increase with age. "Right now, approximately five million Americans over the age of 65 have Alzheimer's, and one in three Americans age 85 and older has Alzheimer's." Dr. Emanuel believes the prospect of that changing in the next few decades is not good and indicates that mental deterioration is a simple function of years. "Even if we aren't demented, our mental functioning deteriorates as we grow older."[7]

Our research points consistently to unhealthy behavior over time as the greater problem. Being a rare genetic "outlier" is not the only reason someone may have greatly increased odds of living a long and far healthier life. Healthy behaviors dramatically change individual prospects. A study of 2,235 men over 35 years found that individuals that practiced at least four out of five healthy behaviors—engaging in regular exercise, not smoking, maintaining a healthy body weight and diet, and consuming low amounts of alcohol—had a 60 percent decrease in dementia and cognitive decline. Exercise was the most powerful mitigating factor. That was just part of the good news. The good-behavior group also enjoyed 70 percent fewer instances of diabetes, heart disease, and stroke than those with consistently poor behavior profiles.[8]

Dr. Emanuel believes that by age 75, creativity, originality, and productivity are pretty much gone for the vast majority of us. "We are subject to who we have been. It is difficult, if not impossible, to generate new, creative thoughts."[9]

This may be the status quo, but it is a consequence of a growing epidemic of bad habits, unhealthy diets, and sedentary lifestyles.

Dr. Emanuel believes we need more research on Alzheimer's, the growing disabilities of old age, and chronic conditions—not on prolonging the dying process. His purpose in sharing his views on old age is to help us think about how we want to live as we grow older. He wants us "to think of an alternative to succumbing to that slow constriction of activities and aspirations imperceptibly imposed by aging."[10] In a nutshell, Dr. Emanuel's advice boils down to this: Please pass the hemlock. He is saying that he hopes to die at 75 and advocates this as a horizon beyond which human life is not worth actively pursuing. He is right about something very important: His observations are a good summary of the wreckage sarcopenia will make of our lives if we do not know and adhere to the remedy—the incredible restorative health benefits of resistance training supported by good nutrition and the avoidance of onerous habits like smoking, alcohol abuse, and abusing drugs.

But, to our surprise, Dr. Emanuel seems not to have read the medical research regarding an alternative to rotting away in place as he imagines. Indeed, he is condescending toward the possibility that exercise has the power to prevent the doom and gloom he sees as an inevitable part of aging: "Americans seem to be obsessed with exercising, doing mental puzzles, consuming various juice and protein concoctions . . . I think this manic desperation to endlessly extend life is misguided and potentially destructive."[11]

Imagine Fred today, as he writes this in Vail, having just finished a day of racing down the most challenging and exhilarating ski slopes with his highly athletic 13-year-old granddaughter, Sophie, reading the warning of a fabulous American medical leader like Dr. Emanuel that his still vigorous, joyful life is something others should not aspire to because doing so is "misguided and potentially destructive."

We used to wonder, and we are sure you are now wondering, how can it be that there is a problem seriously affecting hundreds of millions of people that is so little known and understood outside a small cadre of medical scientists? How has it come to pass that a leading medical bioethicist has concluded that it is best to plan to let go of life after the age of 75? That there is no alternative to long, slow mental and physical deterioration, so we might as well give up, die quickly of pneumonia when it shows up to take us by forgoing antibiotics, and get it all over with? Dr. Emanuel tells us frankly that his personal plan includes refusing antibiotics if he contracts pneumonia once he turns 75.

Now the meaning of the subtitle of his essay becomes crystal clear: "An Argument That Society and Families—and You—Will Be Better Off if Nature Takes Its Course Swiftly and Promptly."[12]

DR. FIELDING ON PREVENTION

Finally, we asked Dr. Roger Fielding, one of the world's leading experts on sarcopenia whom we consulted, why doctors know little about how to prevent sarcopenia. Dr. Fielding explained that there is no medical school that includes courses in exercise physiology or nutrition as part of its MD degree program, and sarcopenia was not given its own International Classification of Diseases code until October 1, 2016.

Dr. Fielding states, "Older patients need to know the problem they have getting up the stairs is because of loss of muscle," he said. "They know about arthritis and high blood pressure, but they don't know that loss of muscle function is not some normal consequence of aging."[13] As an example of how important muscle mass is to life and health, Dr. Fielding told us that "muscle mass is predictive of the number of days a serious cancer patient will survive." The greater the muscle mass, the longer the life.

He also said that resistance exercise is particularly effective for the elderly and that gains in strength of 200 percent are not uncommon once they undertake the specific programs that he and his colleagues recommend. Mobility can be restored to a great many older adults that inactivity has largely immobilized. Dr. Fielding taught us that a rule of thumb about pursuing weight loss through diet without exercise is that 30 percent of the weight lost will be lean (bone and muscle) mass that will never be rebuilt without proper exercise rehabilitation and nutrition that effectively supports lean mass regeneration.

There is progress and a growing effort to tackle this medical condition that to date has largely flown under the radar. Currently, a variety of press reports are introducing the subject of sarcopenia, so a Google search will provide lots of information, and our website, Strongpath.com, acts as a hub for related in-depth news on the subject.

Dr. Fielding believes that prevention is key. Loss of muscle mass over time is a near-universal condition due to sedentary modern lifestyles. Since the condition may advance gradually over the years, most do not realize they are suffering from dangerous and unnecessary muscle wasting until they are overtaken with debilitating weakness. Changing this trend is key to everyone's health and welfare, and the earlier in life the good habits of maintaining muscle health are established, the better.

WHEN DOCTORS FAIL TO ADVISE PREVENTION

It is worthwhile at this point to harken back once again to the fate to which medical science consigns older folks. Baby boomers still mistakenly adhere to worthless slogans like "you are as young as you feel." A 2012 study revealed that "in 2010, only one in three patients who saw a physician in the past 12 months had been advised to exercise or do other physical activity."[14] Vague recommendations like "be active" get mixed with cautions like "not to overdo it," leaving patients to fend for themselves.

Doctors must first learn themselves, and then teach patients, to forget mistaken past conventional wisdom like "take it easy" as key to enjoying life as they age. According to Dr. Travis Saunders, everyone needs to know that most of the severe health impacts of "aging" are not due to aging at all, but to inactivity.[15]

Even though strength training keeps people physically sound and out of nursing homes, few older people do much of it. According to the CDC, in 2012, of those age 75 and over, only 7.9 percent engage in aerobic and strength training that met 2008 federal physical activity guidelines for their age group.[16]

Keep Elders Moving!

According to Dr. Saunders, "We are currently killing our elders with kindness." We worry that perhaps it would be better if they didn't go up and down stairs at their age, even if they seem to be managing them without a problem. We fear that if they go for a walk alone they might not immediately get help if something happens. To placate our own concerns, we encourage them to withdraw too soon from the very activities of daily life that are crucial for their continued wellbeing. Dr. Saunders suggests that we picture the healthiest senior citizen that we know and ask ourselves a question. Does he spend his day "sitting down or walking, skiing, or dancing? It's not a coincidence."[17]

The little-known truth is that if we made a healthy young person sit all day, he would age very rapidly. In a week, his metabolism would collapse and fats would increase. It is inactivity, not aging, that drives the "problems of aging."[18]

Get Up and Stay Up

Inactivity begets more inactivity. This in turn reduces fitness and makes being active even more difficult so that activity levels decrease further. And on and on, as less activity drives more weakness, which drives less fitness in a vicious, declining spiral![19]

The sad end is that even the most successful and accomplished men and women finish their lives in this state of decline. Typical is this recent "end of days" reminiscence by Fay Vincent, born in 1938 and former commissioner of Major League Baseball: "To me, old age seems to be the art of keeping going. Speed and direction are not important. Movement is. I swim, but slowly. I barely walk. I write, but with acute knowledge that my values and opinions are outdated. . . . I want only to be at peace and in normal discomfort. Age makes life simple until it does not. . . . Yes, the rearview mirror is where I get the most pleasure. There I can run and jump and shag high fly balls in the many sunny baseball fields of my youth. There are still those joyful memories of good times and old pals and long-dead family and friends. That is what is left now and that has to be fine with me."[20]

Fred is 10 years older than Mr. Vincent. Fred knows it does not have to be that way. But, without the correct advice from our medical professionals, this will continue to be an accurate description of the downward spiral of weakness and inactivity.

AS WE BEGAN our research into sarcopenia, attending conferences and speaking with medical professionals, most people focused on treating patients toward the end of the death spiral of inactivity instead of teaching them how to prevent this deteriorated state through strength training. The world is facing an epidemic of strength deterioration, and neither the most successful, best-educated people in the world nor their doctors know a thing about it.

Unfortunately, doctors are trained to ensure survival but are not trained to deal with patients' functional abilities; they are not taught exercise physiology or geriatrics. Loss of muscle function is not some normal consequence of aging. Changing the trend is key to everyone's health and welfare, and the earlier in life the good habits of maintaining muscle health are established, the better. Scores of chronic illnesses will follow a sedentary lifestyle like dominoes. And once frailty hits a person, absent targeted interventions, it will get worse with age. The next chapter will reveal just how much of an impact strength training can have on your overall health and how many hideous diseases can be prevented by hitting the gym.

Loss of muscle function is not some normal consequence of aging. Changing the trend is key to everyone's health and welfare, and the earlier in life the good habits of maintaining muscle health are established, the better.

CHAPTER 6

The Remedy: Intense Physical Activity

IN MARCH 2016, Fred and his son were skiing in Vail on one of the best snow days in 40 years. As they drove home, Fred's son said, "Dad, you skied today 30 percent better than you have in the past 45 years. You had way more endurance and strength than I have ever seen before." Exposing our bodies through exercise to the intense physical activity we were designed for is a remedy for the strength loss of sarcopenia. But it is you, not us, who are faced with the decision of staying on the comfortable, familiar Frail Trail or making a life-altering decision to choose the StrongPath. You are likely not comfortable with imposing a hard physical regime on your body based solely on the personal experience of two men, so we are going to share some documented case studies with you at the end of this and other chapters to further inspire you.

You now understand that our bodies were not designed for a sedentary world. To the contrary, the preponderance of favorable

> Exposing our bodies through exercise to the intense physical activity we were designed for is a remedy for the strength loss of sarcopenia.

adaptations in our genes were selected for success in a very different world: a world of comparatively intense daily physical activity. According to developing evolutionary perspectives on disease, as our world became far more sedentary, for the most part in very recent times, our genes—and our bodies—were no longer well matched with our very different modern diets and low levels of activity.

As this mismatch developed and life spans lengthened, so too developed many chronic diseases that have become more prevalent, as has the condition of sarcopenia.[1]

It is noted in physiology journals that chronic diseases that were virtually nonexistent in developing countries are becoming more common as their populations adopt modern diets and become more sedentary. While today's trained athletes may exhibit muscle mass similar to that of our ancient ancestors, and 70-year-olds who continue to engage in challenging exercise can remain robust, modern humans as they age are now characterized more often by "a striking sarcopenia."[2]

Accordingly, our quest now takes us to the question of whether leaving the sedentary path and returning our bodies to intense physical activity can alleviate sarcopenia. In this chapter, we'll examine the science behind why regaining your strength with intense physical activity is critical to reversing sarcopenia and improving your overall health.

SCIENTIFIC RESEARCH, SARCOPENIA, AND STRENGTH TRAINING

Let's take a look at what medical science has learned in recent years regarding whether resistance-training exercise can remedy the lifetime strength-destroying impact of sarcopenia. It is remarkable that sarcopenia research and analysis is still a very new aspect of medical science. Only in the past few years has this disease become an increasingly urgent subject of academic discussion in journals and conferences. As we will see, this important subject remains almost unknown to most physicians. In fact, the first major collection of research and discussion papers was assembled only a few years ago in 2012[3] by Dr. Alfonso Jose Cruz-Jentoft, an expert in geriatric medicine in Spain, titled *Sarcopenia.*

The bottom line in this text is that the logical assumptions we have shared with you are accurate and, in fact, grounded in science. Because muscular atrophy can be caused by inactivity, it makes sense to take our bodies back to the world they were designed for with intense resistance exercise (commonly known as "weight training," "resistance training," or "strength training").

According to Dr. Cruz-Jentoft, the key to keeping our strength as we age is engaging in regular weight training. He explains, "RE [resistance exercise] may be considered the primary preventive or treatment strategy in the battle against sarcopenia."[4] So this specific type of exercise not only helps prevent the loss in muscle strength but can also help to treat and reverse this disease.

THE UNDENIABLE EVIDENCE FOR WEIGHT TRAINING

In his seminal textbook, *Sarcopenia,* Dr. Cruz-Jentoft outlines the concrete scientific evidence that weight training cures this strength-destroying epidemic. He argues that the cheapest and most effective measure to counteract both sarcopenia and osteoporosis is exercise. Studies reveal that a smaller arm circumference, arm muscle circumference, and arm muscle area are related to an increased mortality risk in older men and women.[5] Therefore, increasing the strength and size of these muscles can prolong our longevity.

Dr. Cruz-Jentoft reports the following:

- High-intensity resistance training appears to be most appropriate in dealing with sarcopenia, especially among the old.

- Weight training should be encouraged, regardless of age.

- Age-related loss of strength in severe sarcopenia is detrimental to daily activities and results in physical disability.

- Weight training is excellent protection against age-related loss of strength.

- High-intensity weight training is the best remedy for age-related loss of strength.

THE MEDICAL COMMUNITY

By now, you must be thinking, *If it is so clear and obvious from the leading treatise that weight training is the cure, why did Fred and Steven think it was necessary to write a book about it?* The fact is that, to our total amazement, very few doctors seem to have any understanding of how to cure their patients' insidious loss of strength and mobility. They have repeatedly said, "Frailty with age is inevitable." Apparently, they have never taken the time to learn they are wrong. Our book is critical because there is a huge public and personal health problem that is ruining large parts of people's lives—and the medical community may be largely oblivious to it. Someone has to ring the alarm. With this book, we are undertaking that task.

WE NOW KNOW that sarcopenia caused by inactivity can be remedied by weight training and other physical activity of adequate intensity.

Scientific research by leading doctors in the field of geriatrics has revealed that resistance training along with a diet supporting muscle health are among the most powerful tools for treatment in the battle against sarcopenia. Unfortunately, few doctors seem to understand that this type of physical activity can cure their patients' loss of strength and mobility. In the next section, we'll explore the health benefits of exercise on sarcopenia.

INTENSE EXERCISE HAS INNUMERABLE HEALTH BENEFITS

Forty-eight percent of people who exercise do so for appearance reasons—thinking more about the short-term gains than the long-term ones. The remainder exercise for health reasons, and science has shown that exercise leads to exercisers just plain living longer than sedentary folks. If you are a fit and metabolically healthy obese individual, your risk of all-cause mortality is 38 percent lower than your similarly obese but unfit peers. More startling is the fact that your risk profile is about the same as metabolically healthy individuals of normal weight.[6]

> Scientific research by leading doctors in the field of geriatrics has revealed that resistance training along with a diet supporting muscle health are among the most powerful tools for treatment in the battle against sarcopenia.

Why? Because sedentary lifestyles lead to serious declines in fitness: Muscles atrophy and arteries stiffen, so that people who are more physically active live longer and age better than those who are sedentary. As you're probably now realizing, resistance training is not only important in addressing sarcopenia after it develops into its severe forms. It is critical as a fundamental component of a powerfully preventive lifestyle measure that should be adopted generally for the sake of good health.

In this section, we'll take a look at some of the many chronic diseases that respond well to resistance training, including diabetes, heart disease, cancer, and Alzheimer's. We'll also dispel the myth that your genes hold all the power. They don't. Even if you have a genetic marker for a disease and are more susceptible than others, active intervention through resistance training may have an important impact on your outcome and ability to live a long, healthy life.

THE DEADLY DISEASES OF SEDENTARY BEHAVIOR

Chronic diseases and their accompanying physical ailments take much of the enjoyment out of the last decades of our lives, ruining our remaining days. You are exposing yourself to a shockingly long list of these deadly health issues and chronic diseases by not doing resistance training. Intense exercise can impact mental diseases as well, such as Alzheimer's, panic attacks, and anxiety. Many popular publications are now calling intense exercise the best medicine there is for literally scores of other serious ailments that plague our lives.

Let's think about Dr. Lieberman's "mismatch hypothesis" for a moment and our genome competing in a sedentary world for which it was not designed. We initially began this analysis because we were curious about the possible cause of the epidemic of muscle wasting that has affected almost everyone in the world. Now let's investigate whether there are other diseases besides sarcopenia afflicting us today that were not around 50,000 years ago. It turns out that there are several serious chronic diseases today that seem not to have existed 50,000 years ago. For example, type 2 diabetes, heart disease, osteoporosis, and colon cancer were either absent or much less common for most of our evolutionary history.[7]

If, as we have seen, many other diseases have now become more prevalent, it appears likely that our bodies are not genetically designed to perform well in sedentary conditions. Today, life expectancies are longer than ever, and this gives our bodies ever more opportunity to waste away due to long sedentary years for which our bodies were not intended. Accordingly, it is likely that a highly active physical life with adequate intensity is fundamental to maintaining health and physiological function throughout the entire human life span.

The good news is we can counter or possibly prevent the following chronic diseases by doing intense exercise:

- Diabetes

- Heart disease

- Cancer

- Osteoporosis

- Peripheral artery disease

- Alzheimer's and dementia

Diabetes

It is likely that the most common endocrine disease affecting America today is diabetes. The scale and growth rate of diabetes are both frightening. Type 2 diabetes is caused by factors that include excessive weight that destabilizes our metabolic systems. After we eat, glucose, a form of sugar our bodies use for fuel, enters our bloodstream. Our pancreas then releases insulin, which enables us to use this sugar. Diabetes damages our ability to use the sugar for energy and growth. Instead, excess glucose is stored in the liver. The result can be a long list of awful complications: glaucoma, amputations, kidney disease, heart disease, stroke, nerve damage, increased vulnerability to infections, and more.

Diabetes is now epidemic in the United States. There are more than 26 million diabetics in the United States, and the number is increasing rapidly. Being overweight is the leading risk factor for type 2 diabetes. Two-thirds of Americans are overweight or obese. There are now almost 100 million obese people in the United States, resulting in more than $150 billion a year in additional health costs and an estimated 300,000 deaths a year.[8]

In Hispanic and African-American populations, obesity respectively affects 42 percent and 48 percent of the population. One-third of Caucasians are now obese, and rates are increasing significantly.[9]

Strength training reduces the risk and seriousness of this disease by improving blood sugar control. Increased muscle from weight training helps soak up excess blood sugar, works to store the glucose until needed for fuel, and disperses it when necessary. According to a report in *The Wall Street Journal* by Jen Murphy titled "Managing Diabetes Risk with Diet and Exercise,"[10] keeping muscle fibers strong and active is important for their protective effect. It is no surprise, therefore, that exercise can help prevent type 2 diabetes and may even reverse the disease. For example, 10 diabetic Australian Aborigines returned to a high-exercise, hunter-gatherer lifestyle. After 7 weeks, the diet and exercise had almost entirely reversed their diabetes.[11]

> Exercise can help prevent type 2 diabetes and may even reverse the disease.

It is important to note that both cardio and strength training are valuable in fighting diabetes, but according to a 2016 article in *The*

Wall Street Journal, "If you only have time for one, choose resistance training."[12]

Heart Disease

Heart disease is the primary health risk in the United States, according to the Cleveland Clinic.[13] Despite all we hear about cancer, heart disease remains the top killer of both men and women. Surprisingly, heart disease is "a lifestyle disease" that is preventable in the vast majority of cases. According to Steven Nissen, MD, of the Cleveland Clinic, "If you know your risk factors and if you pay attention to them, this is a disease that we do know how to prevent."[14] We can modify the risk factors—increase activity, decrease excess body fat, and control issues like high cholesterol, high blood pressure, and diabetes. Modifying our lifestyle helps, and all of these things respond favorably to strength training.[15]

It's not just our theory either. The chief of cardiovascular medicine at Cleveland Clinic[16] says that the evidence is remarkable that exercise—

- Lowers blood pressure

- Sharply raises good cholesterol

- Improves blood vessel functioning

- Forms new blood vessels

- Reduces blood clots in coronary arteries

Indeed, the New York State Department of Health says, "It is estimated that approximately 35% of coronary heart disease mortality is due to physical inactivity."[17] Dr. Nissen says that "vigorous exercise has a therapeutic effect as good as any drug. . . . It reduces the risk of disease . . . improves cognition and the quality of life." He is clear in his conclusion: Exercise is medication—better than anything we have.[18]

There are large, well-controlled studies revealing that unfit Americans can cut their risk of heart disease in half simply by exercising. And think about this: Data from 2011 suggests that persuading just 25 percent of unfit Americans to exercise would save $58 billion a year in health-care costs later,[19] which is nearly twice what the National Institutes of Health (NIH) invested in medical research in 2016.

Doctors Are Catching On, but Slowly

Knowledge of muscles and the full role they play in human health is in its infancy. Human heath depends on muscle health. Yet sarcopenia was not even recognized with an International Classification of Diseases code until October 2016. The failure to recognize this life-threatening malady sooner with a simple official diagnostic code meant that even the few doctors who knew about the devastating effects of sarcopenia had difficulty treating the condition and getting paid by insurers for their effort.

According to Dr. Nissen at the Cleveland Clinic, doctors are just beginning to appreciate all the spillover effects and the power of strength training to remedy and prevent heart disease.

In fact, the American Heart Association recommends strength training at least twice per week. But what if you have had a heart attack or stroke? The National Institute of Aging says, "Some people are afraid to exercise after a heart attack. But regular physical activity can help reduce your chances of having another heart attack."[20] The American Heart Association also published a statement in 2014 saying that "doctors should prescribe exercise to stroke patients, since there is strong evidence that physical activity and exercise after stroke can improve cardiovascular fitness, walking ability, and upper arm strength."[21]

The American Heart Association cautions that "if you've had a heart attack or stroke, you should talk with your doctor before starting any exercise to be sure you're following a safe, effective physical activity program."[22]

Many cardiologists are willing to extend their prescription of exercise as a medicine even further. People who have had heart attacks may start strength training as few as 3 weeks after the attack if their cardiologists recommend it, rather than waiting the more conservative 4–6 months proposed in older guidelines.

Cancer

Dr. Fielding explained to us that strength and muscle mass can be predictive of how long we survive cancer. The research we've gathered suggests that there are multiple ways in which strength training and physical activity can affect varying types of cancer. Some of these are surprising. For example, a 2009 study[23] included 8,677 men ages 20–82 and followed them from 1980 to 2003. It looked primarily at all-cause cancer mortality. This long-term study produced three main findings. First, greater muscle strength was associated with lower cancer mortality risk in men, independent of confounding factors such as age, smoking, alcohol consumption, and health status. Second, higher body fat percentages and larger waist circumference were associated with higher cancer mortality rates. No surprise there, but the association did not persist for those in this group with greater strength and better cardiovascular fitness. Third, cancer mortality rates were 40–50 percent higher in the group consisting of the lower third in terms of muscular strength with high adiposity.

How can greater strength and better fitness possibly help fight cancer? This question places us right on the frontier of research, and recent findings are tantalizingly beginning to reveal mechanics operating at the genetic level. At a 2012 meeting of the American Society of Clinical Oncology in San Francisco, a University of California–San Francisco research team presented a study that looked at twenty thousand genes in the healthy portion of the tissue of men with low-grade prostate cancer. Amazingly, they were able to identify 184 genes whose expression (actively producing a protein product) in the prostate gland is linked to vigorous exercise. Among the genes that were more active were the well-known "tumor suppressor" genes BRCA1 and BRCA2, as well as other genes known to be involved in DNA repair.[24] Disease-specific research linking adequate exercise to improved health is substantial and growing.

Colon Cancer

There has been more research on the relationship between colon cancer and physical activity than most other cancers.[25] There is convincing evidence that those who increase the intensity of their physical activity reduce their risk of getting colon cancer. The mechanisms of the protection are still under investigation, but the fact of the protection provided by adequately intense exercise is undisputed.

And it's not just prevention. Participants of physical activity experienced enhanced survival *after* a cancer diagnosis. We feel that as the medical community is better able to study and research the impact of varying exercise intensity levels, more important details will be revealed about the relationship between colon cancer and physical activity.

Breast Cancer

In *The Ecology of Breast Cancer: The Promise of Prevention and the Hope for Healing* by Ted Schettler MD, MPH,[26] we learn that the effect that physical activity has on breast cancer has also been long studied. In this section, we will cover some of the critical points you should know. For example, most studies show that active women (particularly post-menopausal women) have a lower risk of developing breast cancer. The amount that breast cancer risk is reduced through activity ranges from 20–80 percent. The range is broad, because an individual's risk profile goes up or down depending on many factors. Starting exercise early in life is a big plus. Women under 45 who were not college athletes are more than 6 times as likely to suffer breast cancer than those who were college athletes. What about all women of any age that never were high-caliber athletes, but have been active? An analysis of more than 40,000 women by the Nurses' Health Study II[27] revealed that those with lifetime patterns of exercise decreased the risk of developing conditions that increase the growth of certain cells in the breast that are generally considered an early stage in developing breast cancer.

Endometrial Cancer

There have been thirty-three research studies as of this writing on physical activity and endometrial cancer. These studies indicate a reduced risk of 6–30 percent, depending on the forms of physical activity studied. The mechanism for the benefit is thought to be changes in body mass and in levels of sex hormones.[28]

Lung Cancer

A May 2016 meta-analysis of eighteen studies showed that former and current smokers benefited from recreational physical activity. Both groups were shown to have a 23 percent reduced risk of contracting the disease.[29]

Prostate Cancer

There is exciting new research regarding the role of exercise in the mortality of prostate cancer patients. A study concludes that more physical activity has a protective effect from both death from cancer and, surprisingly, death from any cause at all. One of the studies even quantifies the protective effect: 61 percent less chance of death from cancer for those that are physically active and 46 percent less chance of dying from any cause when cancer patients pick up the pace and are physically active at a moderate to intense level.[30]

Another study suggested "that regular vigorous activity could slow the progression of prostate cancer" in men age 65 or older.[31] This study, which also reviewed data from over 1,000 actual cases of prostate cancer, observed an overall 54 percent risk reduction, and a 69 percent risk reduction in older men, in metastatic prostate cancer.

The (Literally) Killer Potbelly

The first time Fred ever thought about potbellies was when he noticed a slogan over the door of the gymnasium at West Point: "A Pot Belly Cannot Lead Men." This was enough for him. The problem with a potbelly is that it has much more serious health issues than simply looking bad.

Fat accumulated in the glutes, thighs, and lower body (the pear shape) is subcutaneous, while deeper fat in the abdominal area (the apple shape) is largely visceral. Subcutaneous fat is largely located just under the skin but there is emerging evidence that the danger of big potbellies lie in both deep visceral and subcutaneous fat. Visceral fat is found deep within the abdominal cavity where it fills the spaces between our abdominal organs.

What causes a relatively slender person to grow a potbelly lapping over his or her belt? It has to do with how our bodies evolved to succeed in a dangerous, intense world. The fight-or-flight response, up to somewhere between 30,000 and 70,000 years ago by current estimates, was all about facing life-and-death threats in reality. During this period, something new began to happen. Humans underwent a cognitive revolution. We began to mentally envision ourselves and imagine. With imagination came self-reflection and worry.

Our bodies selected for characteristics useful for dealing with threats and preparing our bodies to fight or flee from a threat. A cascade of hormones is triggered that increases our blood pressure and blood sugar and suppresses our immune system. This provides a boost of energy while other hormones, such as adrenaline, support immediate violent muscular action.

Of course, today, we often feel stress and fear about things that have not actually occurred and may never occur. Nevertheless, this still releases all these substances because our brain tells us we are going to have to fight or flee. Unlike our prehistoric ancestors responding to actual immediate threats, we rarely actually fight or flee from a threat. A worry just lingers in our minds for long periods of time. We also experience a stress response because of work deadlines, which might cause our boss to be angry, or we fret about an imagined threat and embarrassment that might cause us to lose status. When stressed, we experience repeated concerns over things that do not call for physical fighting or fleeing. Because of this, the fatty acids we emitted for energy to fight or flee a threat are unused and accumulate in the abdomen, producing a world-class potbelly.

Now, from a health point of view, is there a difference between gluteal fat and abdominal fat? Gluteal fat, while unsightly, sits below our skin and does not surround any vital organs. We may not like how it looks, but it is much less threatening to our health than abdominal or visceral fat, which is a major cause of many serious health problems.

Visceral fat is chemically active, leaking dangerous chemicals to our internal organs. As a result, according to Harvard Health Publications, visceral fat is linked to metabolic disturbances. These occur when an abnormal chemical reaction disrupts the balance and functioning of hormones. Visceral fat also increases the risk for cardiovascular disease and type 2 diabetes.[32]

Visceral fat yields to regular physical activity of significant intensity and strength training. These should be combined with a sensible diet featuring portion control, fresh fruits, vegetables, and lean proteins in place of simple carbohydrates to bring dangerous visceral fat under control.[33]

Peripheral Artery Disease

More than eight million Americans have trouble even walking because of diseased or blocked arteries in their legs.[34] Their resulting avoidance of walking makes them sedentary and more likely to be obese and suffer from myriad other conditions. Worse, the number of people suffering from peripheral artery disease is rapidly increasing. This disease is underdiagnosed and undertreated. Because the disease makes it painful to walk, this appears odd indeed. The reason is people either adapt to the disease by not walking or think it is a normal consequence of aging.

It turns out a first treatment for this disease is supervised exercise. The prescription is walking until it hurts. Note the time walked.

Rest until the pain subsides. Then start again and walk until the pain returns. Continue this until the total time spent just walking adds up to 20–30 minutes. This drill causes exercise tolerance to build up as supplemental blood vessels form in the legs. This prescription of exercise results in patients being able to walk long distances without pain.[35]

Life-Ending Bone Fractures

Most of us are oblivious to the problem of the life-ending bone fractures facing all of us as we age. Sure, we remember Aunt Helen, who fell down when she was 70, became bedridden, and just faded away and died in a few years. But the cause of these terrible events, and the cure, are not on our radar screens. We never think about them, do we? So just what is this largely ignored and little-known issue?

> Two pounds of muscle are lost by just 10 days in a hospital.

The track is a simple one. Falls lead to fractures and 87 percent of hip fractures specifically result from falls. Increased leisure, sports, and chores and reduced daily periods of inactivity correlate with a significantly reduced risk for hip fracture. But the aging population is ever more sedentary. So a third of elderly people fall each year, and 10–15 percent of those result in fracture,[36] which leads to prolonged bedrest, which causes a further loss of strength, bone, and muscle mass, leading to further injury. Two pounds of muscle are lost by just 10 days in a hospital for otherwise healthy older adults.[37] Once that muscle and bone is gone, the falls come faster, and we become trapped in the fatal downward spiral. According to International Osteoporosis Foundation, "Almost 60% of those who fell the previous year will fall again."[38] The remedy for this, of course, is physical therapy that strengthens lower limbs and makes them more capable.

Harvard Medical School on Bone Loss

"Numerous studies have shown that strength training can play a role in slowing bone loss, and several show it can even build bone. This is tremendously useful to help offset age-related decline in bone mass, especially among postmenopausal women."[39]

Alzheimer's and Dementia

Alzheimer's is likely the most dreaded disease among baby boomers. Whenever we raise the subject of Alzheimer's in a group of boomers, they always change the subject. Our impression is that it is the disease no one wants to discuss or learn much about—nor do people want to know if they have the gene tied to the disease.

There is no mystery regarding why Alzheimer's is so feared. It is a conscious, slow spiraling into a living death. It is accompanied by a stark awareness that all that makes us human is sifting through our fingers, with every hour being lived in an awareness of facing the worst doom imaginable—a loss of mental competence and conscious awareness of relationships with loved ones.

Researchers suspect that Alzheimer's insidiously begins to shrink parts of our brains, including those essential to memory processing. In our 50s, that part of the brain shrinks by 1–2 percent a year. Scans of brains of Alzheimer's victims show considerable shrinkage compared to people the same age without Alzheimer's. Most of us experience some cognitive decline and many develop Alzheimer's.[40]

If there were a drug that could be taken beginning in our 50s that had a 60 percent chance of preventing brain shrinkage and Alzheimer's, it would be the most valuable drug in history. Even if it cost $10,000 a year, everyone who could afford the drug would take it.

Alzheimer's has been described as a pandemic disease. Between 2000 and 2013, deaths from Alzheimer's increased 71 percent. A real cure would be huge. Guess what? There is something as good or better than existing expensive Alzheimer's drugs. And it is free.

> Those who expend the most energy exercising are 90 percent less likely to develop cognitive decline.

And almost no one, including your doctors, knows what the preventive remedy is. It's called exercise. "For the past few years, physical exercise [a minimum of three 30-minute sessions per week] has been as good or better than anything that we can recommend for people with or at risk for cognitive decline," writes Samuel Gandy, the director of the Mount Sinai Center for Cognitive Health and NFL Neurological Center[41]

Huge numbers of Americans will experience the terrible, conscious, knowing spiral down into loss of all that counts in life. And many will learn in the middle of the spiral that there was a preventive remedy that no one told them about: exercise. Exercise is the most significant protection against Alzheimer's. Those who expend the most energy exercising are 90 percent less likely to develop cognitive decline.[42] And just 1 hour of exercise per week cuts the chances of getting Alzheimer's in half.[43]

The hard evidence for intense exercise is extensive:

- According to a recent study in *The Journal of the American Geriatrics Society*, women who had white matter brain lesions that did resistance training twice a week for a year had significantly lower white matter lesion volume at the end of the study than those who did balance and tone exercise twice a week.[44]

- According to the BBC, a study spanning 35 years by Cardiff

University found that exercise throughout a person's life plays a significant role in reducing the risk of developing dementia. Exercise was the single biggest influence on dementia levels of the five factors studied.[45]

- According to nature.com, "There is now strong evidence that links regular physical activity or exercise to higher cognitive function, decreased cognitive decline, and reduced risk of AD [Alzheimer's disease] or dementia."[46] According to Dr. J. Eric Ahlskog in the Department of Neurology at the Mayo Clinic in Rochester, Minnesota: "You can make a very compelling argument for exercise as a disease-modifying strategy to prevent dementia and mild cognitive impairment, and for favorably modifying these processes once they have developed."[47]

Exercise Can Trump Bad Genes

Even those with a genetic predisposition for developing Alzheimer's can use exercise to ward off their genetic inheritance. The APOE gene is the only gene known to be related to late-onset Alzheimer's disease. We have two APOE genes, one from our father and one from our mother. The most common are the APOE2, APOE3, or APOE4 variants. Forty percent of all people with late-onset Alzheimer's disease have either one or two APOE4 genes, even though they represent only 25–30 percent of the population.[48]

In a major study, carriers of the APOE4 gene who did little exercise experienced 3 percent shrinkage of part of the brain governing memory in only 18 months. Carriers of the APOE4 who exercised had almost no shrinkage.[49]

According to Stephen M. Rao, a professor at the Schey Center for Cognitive Neuroimaging at the Cleveland Clinic, exercise seems to be protective of the brains of people carrying the APOE4 gene, known to indicate high risk for Alzheimer's.[50]

It's never too late to start. It is much better to start early, but exercise can act as a protective mechanism against Alzheimer's even at advanced ages. A Finnish study revealed the favorable effects of exercise for cognitive decline even at ages 67–77.[51]

EXERCISE IS MEDICINE FOR OUR BRAINS

It is known that exercise creates new mitochondria in the brain cells of mice. Very active mice experience neurogenesis in certain areas of their brains.[52]

But scientists have not known whether exercise also makes existing brain cells fitter the same way they make existing muscles fitter. Where muscles are concerned, experiments have proven that exercise both causes the growth of new muscle mitochondria and improves the vitality of existing mitochondria. Exercise thus drives a "very potent cellular reaction" in our muscles, which leads to endurance and increased longevity in animals.[53]

Brain cells are also fueled by mitochondria—the powerhouses of a cell. But no one had been able to figure out if exercise triggered similar beneficial responses in brain cells. Scans had shown increased metabolic activity in brain cells during workouts, but it was not known if those active brain cells were adapting and changing due to the exercise.

An article in *The New York Times* covered a South Carolina University study that revealed the examination of the brains of exercised and unexercised mice. Tissue samples from the cells of exercising mice showed that their brain cells contained "newborn" mitochondria. There was no similar finding in the sedentary mice. The researchers concluded that 2 months of exercise training for mice could indeed increase mitochondrial biogenesis, which is the production of new living organelles in the brain cells.[54]

This study is revolutionary because it suggests exercise-driven changes in cells other than muscle cells. There are many different exciting possibilities once we understand what this research shows:

- Creating more mitochondria may alleviate neurogenerative diseases like Parkinson's and Alzheimer's.

- Brains energized by more mitochondria may be more resistant to fatigue and able to help the body exercise longer and more vigorously.

- Revitalized brain cells may sharpen thinking.[55]

It seems almost possible that exercise could cure or alleviate the long list of chronic ills we have discussed in this chapter. Our advice to live a life of intense physical exercise would be worth it if only one of these many serious problems were helped. The scientific proof that muscular health and strength is fundamental to health and critical to both the prevention or treatment of chronic diseases ought to clinch the choice you now know looms before you.

THE EXERCISE FIX

There are sensible reasons exercise is so effective across a broad spectrum of chronic diseases. Most of the time, when we discuss the myriad diseases addressed by exercise, our audiences reply with skepticism: "How in the world could lifting weights remedy serious problems, ranging from heart disease to cancer to Alzheimer's?" But the fact is exercise does work for these chronic diseases, most of the time better than medicine.

Remember, it is not just our muscles that were selected for success in a physically active world. It is every cell in our body, from our skin to our brain to our vascular system, that was long ago specifically chosen to compete in a physically active world. The problem is that the world we were designed for no longer exists. Today, our bodies must compete in a world we were not designed for—a totally sedentary world. A relatively new theory holds that our bodies are therefore out of sync with the world in which we now operate. We were made for a different world and are not genetically matched for success in this one.[56]

UNFORTUNATELY, WE CANNOT reengineer our genes to prevent chronic mismatch diseases by tweaking or altering our genome to match today's sedentary environment. Therefore, we must change our environment and lifestyle to better fit our genome. Looked at this way, it is not at all surprising that most of these chronic ills can be cured or remedied in large part by exercise. Exercise puts our bodies back in the world they were made for and helps prevent the disease caused by the mismatch.

Exercise is a frontline approach to prevention of cancer, heart disease, and Alzheimer's and may help suppress low-grade inflammation. And while it's good to start early, scientific evidence reveals that even starting an exercise regime later in life can protect the brain and your ability to survive diseases. So where do you start?

We realize that, for many people, exercise can be intimidating and tough to sustain for the long haul. We don't want you to hit the gym for a month or two and then quit. We want you to make this a habit for life—like brushing your teeth. To accomplish that, you need mental motivation. And we're going to provide that at the end of this chapter with our first case study, where you will meet Peter. In this case study, you will learn how Peter got started on the StrongPath and how he stayed on track. In the chapters that follow, we share new case studies with you to further inspire you as you dive deeper into the StrongPath.

CASE STUDY: PETER

Peter is a 58-year-old software developer who describes himself as a former athlete who has gone to seed. He had pounds to lose and strength and fitness to gain after 15 years of doing no weight training while working at a desk. He had done some heavy lifting in the past, when he had been active with karate from ages 30 to 42, but he had stopped after a change in employment.

Peter had relatively little training before coming into the program, even with his martial arts practice. He experienced strength gains that can only be explained by the initial training adaptations that take place among the generally sedentary population. He certainly developed greater muscle definition while participating in this study, but his level of improvement is more likely attributable to the vast improvements in his overall motor behavior, exercise technique, and neuromuscular activation. Peter improved his technique as a result of this training, and while he started with noticeable shoulder and knee pain, he was able to accomplish his workouts consistently due to improved form with the exercises. On several occasions, we used variations of exercises to reeducate him on the use of certain muscle groups to improve his lifting and reduce his perceived pain. His work to learn how to move more effectively is undoubtedly also responsible for his improvement as evidenced in the chart below.

Fear Factor

Peter went into his initial session terrified. He told us later that he thought he was going to look stupid by being pushed beyond his comfort zone in front of people he knew at the club. He learned something immediately: Everyone there was actually pulling for him. Everyone was pulling for everyone, in fact. The gym isn't full of people who want you to fail. Peter said they all seemed genuinely happy to see other people being active, and they were encouraging to anyone and everyone on their own personal missions. His fears were allayed when he realized no one was looking down at him for starting out and being behind in his fitness status. Those fears had been in his head only.

> " Everyone was pulling for everyone, in fact. The gym isn't full of people who want you to fail.

Biggest Surprise

Peter was astonished by how weak he'd become over the years—a fact that revealed itself during his first few sessions. He'd yo-yo dieted before starting the strength program and kept active with karate, but when he began his sessions with Cullen, he couldn't lift anywhere near what he had 15 years earlier. He couldn't believe how off his balance was. He was also surprised by how good he ultimately felt as he got stronger. He wasn't sure he wanted to be a part of this experiment initially, but as it progressed, he realized it was his opportunity to not only get in physical shape but to also feel good about himself.

Benefits

Aside from the obvious increase in strength (as evidenced in the chart below) and positive shift in physical appearance, Peter noticed that he walks lighter, which he said feels great. He hasn't lost pounds, and would still like to, but he is tighter in general. Peter said he is happier, more alert, and "less disgusted" with his physique. He's not less tired, but he sleeps longer and more soundly after his workouts. "I have no trouble getting to sleep at night," he said. At work, he's seen a profound increase in his mental sharpness. Since he solves problems for a living, he said he's now more effective at doing so. He said his mind is better able to concentrate now that he's physically stronger.

There were added physical benefits beyond the day-to-day, too. "One of my goals is to test for another degree of black belt," he said. "But with my age, the quality of the technique that I can do from experience alone, and just from having done millions and millions of repetitions, I can generate a lot of force inside my body with punches and kicks. However, I am not strong enough to handle that equal and opposite reaction that happens inside the body from generating all that force. In the past, I got injured and pulled muscles all the time. I would get into a bad cycle and be unable to train because I'd injured something. What I really do feel I got out of this training is that I got the body and the muscular strength to be able to handle that force now. And so I'm not injuring myself anymore when I do karate."

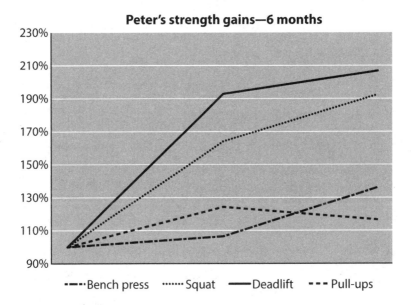

Peter's strength gains—6 months

- ----Bench press   ⋯⋯ Squat   ——Deadlift   - - - Pull-ups

Words of Wisdom

"Welcome your pain," said Peter. He said he used strength training to welcome that pain because it's good pain. It means you're pushing yourself harder each day. "If you're going at it and you're improving yourself," he said, "you are going to be in pain."

Peter's observation about pain is important. Our pain experience is subjective. We actually feel pain more or less intensely depending on whether or not we believe the sensation is signaling damage or benefit.[57] If you come to understand that sore muscles after exercise are a sign of a beneficial process—and that the result of that pain will be increased strength—you'll be better able to change your relationship with pain, and to experience that pain as a positive sensation.

> ❝
>
> **We actually feel pain more or less intensely depending whether or not we believe the sensation is signaling damage or benefit.**

Mind Games: Steven's Solution

> Reality is invariably kinder and fuller of hopeful prospects than our fears would suggest.

Entering an unfamiliar situation, especially among strangers, can inevitably evoke a worried self-consciousness. This form of self-consciousness is the enemy of self-confidence. It's the kind of mental preoccupation that can make us trip over our own feet trying to step onto a stage or cause us to forget our own name when we are overwhelmed by being put on the spot in front of an audience. Don't struggle against it. Giving the rising feeling of panic more attention will not allay your fears. Take a deep breath and go in. Open your senses fully. Concentrate on what your senses are reporting, like Peter did, rather than on the voice in your head, which is prone to catastrophizing. That voice lives in its own world and leaves little attention available for reality. Reality is invariably kinder and fuller of hopeful prospects than our fears would suggest.

There is another interesting aspect about being self-conscious: Attention is a limited resource. I believe that turning attention away from present-moment reality in favor of self-conscious worry decreases the neural activation potential of muscle-cell motor units. I witness in working with people in the gym that the objective weight they can handle declines when their attention is somewhat internally preoccupied. As Tim Gallwey has observed broadly in sports and in life in general, "Performance equals potential minus interference."[58] This seems very true. Being self-conscious amounts to a turning away of attention from movement in real time, and that makes us physically less capable, clumsier, and generally out of step with reality.

One-Year Update

After 12 months on the StrongPath, Peter greatly improved his dead lift. Beginning with a 75-pound dead lift ability, he can now deadlift 235 pounds. He can execute two unassisted body-weight pull-ups using full range of motion and keeping his palms forward. And his bench-press max is now 115 pounds.

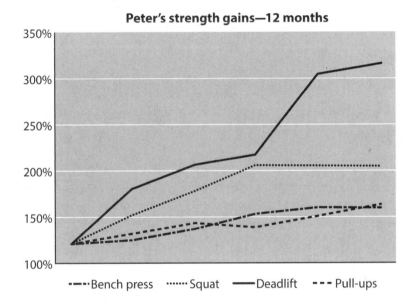

Peter's strength gains—12 months

CHAPTER 7

The Motivation We All Need

SINCE OUR SOLUTION to the downward spiral of sarcopenia involves hard physical work, you might imagine that the primary obstacles to choosing the StrongPath are physical ones. You would be wrong. The reasons so few choose the StrongPath are overwhelmingly mental—the reasons are in our heads.

To understand your mental blocks—your resistance to working out, your resistance to developing good habits—you need to acknowledge them and then learn how to change your mind. In this chapter, we will explain the mental portion of our push to get you on track toward enjoying a healthy, strong life.

OUR BODY AND MIND BUILD EACH OTHER

Fred is by long habit and training a man of action. When he and Steven first met, Fred was averse to considering the "touchy-feely" aspects of things. But, while he did not let common human reactions to difficulties and reversals stop him from acting, Fred still felt all the internal sensations everyone does, such as butterflies in his stomach before an important jury argument or fear when looking down an extremely steep ski slope. As he and Steven talked through what was going on internally that caused these feelings, Fred rapidly began to evolve his personal techniques for dealing with difficulties and reversals into a more broadly applicable working understanding that he now sees as critical to teaching the StrongPath.

Fred has commented that many of his long-term close friends say, "Fred, I know you are right, but I just do not have the willpower to do what is necessary." And these are uniformly hardworking people who have attained great success. So don't beat yourself up if you've been known to have the same defeatist thoughts.

Do know this: It is not unusual or generally unattainable willpower that is the continuing force that keeps Fred on track. So what's Fred's secret? Habit.

Fact

The *Journal of Clinical Psychology* tells us that only 8 percent successfully keep the resolutions they make.[1]

"Habit is far more important than willpower. Willpower, like a bicep, can only exert itself so long before it gives out; it's an extremely limited mental resource."[2] Fred has learned to utilize the weak force of willpower to efficiently establish the strong and durable force of habit. This allows him to act consistently over time in accord with important things he has learned. We will address this process in detail later in this chapter. Once you understand the science and the reality, your initial resistance will dissolve as the path ahead opens up, first mentally and then physically.

> **The StrongPath is as much a mental transformation as it is a physical one.**

Few, if any, begin with the good habits and beneficial attitudes that were Fred's, and that is why he could find his way to the StrongPath initially. But good habits and attitudes were not his from birth. He learned them from his mother, Agnes; his wife, Jana; and from his life experience. And you can learn them, too. The StrongPath is as much a mental transformation as it is a physical one. Habits of thought can easily defeat us even before we get started, so it is important to address them from the very beginning.

Fact

"Habits can comprise cognitive expressions of routine (habits of thought) as well as motor expressions of routine."[3]

As time passes, we get set in our ways. This is a way of saying much of behavior and attitude is habitual. We do what we have always done; we say what we have always said. Long-standing sedentary behavior patterns and avoidance of challenging exercise become a collection of habits that we are comfortable with, even though they are ruinous to our health.

As we decline physically, getting weaker and less capable with each passing year, a sense of inevitability grows. This is exacerbated as we see our ability to function in the normal activities of life steadily eroding. Over time, a feeling of certainty that there is little or nothing that can be done differently takes hold, and hopelessness can flood over us.

Physical decline, therefore, goes hand in hand with a decline in self-image: how you picture yourself in your mind. It is important to remember that this self-image is imaginary, not fixed, although it may seem so at any given moment. It is a big stew composed of some current information and lots of past information mixed with feelings and thoughts about yourself and seasoned with sweet dreams and sharp fears concerning what lies ahead.

Your mental image of yourself and your physical body constantly affect and shape each other. Your mental self-image often leads the process of physical formation by internally projecting and producing an influential vision of your future. Few of us appreciate how much mental imaging influences our actual physical health and well-being.

> Your mental self-image often leads the process of physical formation by internally projecting and producing an influential vision of your future.

Research has found that "older individuals with more positive self-perceptions of aging . . . lived 7.5 years longer than those with less positive self-perceptions of aging. This advantage remained after age, gender, socioeconomic status, loneliness, and functional health were included as covariates."[4] This mental factor also proves powerful during times of crisis. For example, older individuals with a positive self-image are 44 percent more likely to fully recover from a severe disability and resume activities of daily living.[5]

None of us are immune and none of us intend to have a negative self-image. In Steven's case, he just thought he was being realistic—and he slipped gradually into being less than he could be slowly over time, punctuated by some dramatic downward slides.

STEVEN'S HEALTH JOURNEY—A DOWNWARD SPIRAL THWARTED

Steven believed that he had physically peaked around his 27th birthday. Around that time, work, which had been much more physical when he was younger, became all about going to an office. By his mid-30s, he found that if he dove for a tennis shot a little out of reach, he no longer bounced and rolled unharmed. He would hurt himself and his friends would say things like "you're not a kid anymore" and "it's hell getting older." While not quite 40, he did notice he was becoming less resilient.

When he reached 45, one of those dramatic slides occurred. He was sitting at his desk one afternoon when he got a call from his dermatologist. He had gone in to have a dime-size mole removed from his right calf. He was told that the lab had determined it to be advanced melanoma and that he was to report to the hospital for surgery ASAP. A few days later, he returned home with about half of his calf removed, and life suddenly became about hobbling around on crutches, injecting interferon, and worrying about surviving cancer.

Over the following months, events had a drastic effect on his self-image and his sense of where life was heading. After 7 months on interferon, his hair was falling out in disturbing patches, he constantly felt sick and tired, and he had to take naps after injections. The face looking back at him from the mirror looked haggard, and then things took another dramatic turn for the worse.

He got a cough that would not go away. It intensified over a few days until it was continuous. He made his way one night to an emergency clinic, and an X-ray showed that he had pneumonia. He was sent to the local emergency room where they confirmed the diagnosis, checked him in, and put him on intravenous antibiotics. His condition continued to deteriorate, and he got an extreme and persistent fever. Ice was packed in bags under his arms and in his groin. He could not eat, drink, or sleep without violently choking. This continued for more than 2 weeks, and his weight dropped from 185 to 145 pounds. Although he was still a young man, his physical body and self-image were collapsing.

His blood was sent to the CDC for fear he had picked up some exotic bug when travelling in Asia or Africa. It came back in time with a diagnosis of valley fever, a pneumonia-causing fungus found in the soil in the southwest United States. Human immune systems usually handle it without getting ill, but Steven's immune system, weakened by interferon, could not cope and his condition had become nearly fatal. His lungs and vocal cords were damaged. He could not speak.

Given Diflucan, which had been approved for use only 6 months earlier, he began to pull through, and in a week he was back home—still unable to speak but breathing, with difficulty, and recovering.

As we learned earlier, accidents and infections ended the lives of most individuals at the turn of the twentieth century without them suffering a long period of disability. The average life span for a male in the United States in 1900 was 46. At the time, Steven was 46. It was 1997, and he had squeaked by thanks to a just-in-time correct medical diagnosis and pharmaceutical advances. If it had been his grandfather or his father, their lives would have been over.

Not yet 50, he felt old, frail, and no longer confident in his health or strength. He was getting better physically, but his self-image had been shaken and had emerged weak and unsure. Intellectually, he was still sound, so he began to rely on that strength and rebuilt his self-image. Otherwise, he was old and needed his rest, his back was weak from long bed rest periods, and it was time to slow down. If a friend needed help moving, forget it. Those days were long gone.

He saw himself in those terms. He accepted this vision of his limitations, and, over time, he physically grew into them and became the image that he saw. He did not believe he had a choice. That was "him" now. He made peace with the idea of greatly reduced physical ability going forward and lived it.

That's when Steven met Fred, who was almost 20 years older than Steven. At the time of this writing, Fred is 85 and continues to be very strong. If he needs to move furniture, no problem.

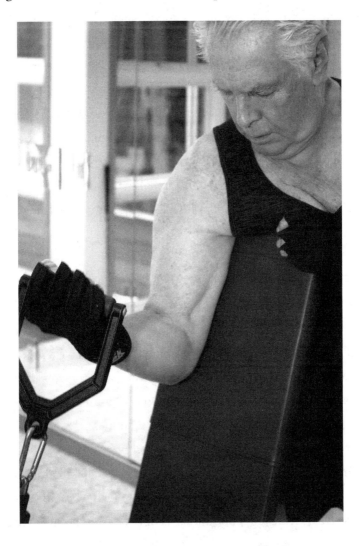

Figure 7.1. Fred Bartlit, 85 and going strong.

Fred challenged Steven's self-image and the assumptions they were based on; he was living proof of a possibility. He was an image of old age Steven had never seen before. But he was an outlier, and Steven figured his health circumstances were different. He was doing what was right for him. He had to be Steven. He could not just morph into a version of Fred. He was not only different from him but also different from everyone else. Right?

The chatter in Steven's head said the same things to him that he now hears being said to Fred by most others. Because of his training, he knows it is a mistake to follow the impulse of the voice in his head. Instead, he shifted his attention and began to envision being strong again, like Fred. He knew it would take a while and that he could not be in a hurry. He was extremely weak and would have to start from where he was, incrementally working to get stronger. He would not be Fred. He would be himself, but Fred allowed him to see a vision of a possible reality, something attainable, something he was missing for lack of trying.

EACH OF US sees our personal story in our own way. Doing so sets a default course of automatic choices that we simply have a predilection to follow. This is its power. Our story is strong and controls most of us, because we do not know how to alter the vision of ourselves that is accepting and expecting a downward spiral of health as we age.

Part of our vision of self has to do with participating in social and class norms that can have a surprising ability to lock us into our circumstances. Many of us have never been involved in strength training because we have never been "that kind of person" or because we didn't know anyone who was.

> ## Fact
>
> Prejudice is also operative in self-image and choice. "Upper middle-class Americans avoid 'excessive displays of strength,' viewing the bodybuilder look as a vulgar overcompensation for wounded manhood."[6]

But if we set any misgivings aside for a moment and allow ourselves to see a new vision, based on a real possibility, then a new path emerges. We cannot change our past, but the present is forever a potential pivot point, and our future begins anew every time we seize an inspiring and practical vision and begin to walk down the path it opens for us.

Steven woke up in a sense from a dark vision he had sunken into while he was sick. He had not walked out of it and regrouped mentally until he met Fred. Soon after, he took the plunge, went to the gym, and started a strength-training program, along the lines Fred had pursued for decades.

A SECOND CHALLENGE EMERGED

Steven is 66 now. Four years ago, his health was seriously challenged again when he had bypass surgery and his chest was opened up, sternum sawn in half. But he was ready to recover this time. He was up walking the halls of the hospital the day after surgery. He was released from the hospital the second day after surgery and kept developing his lower-body strength. After 2 months, he was allowed to begin lifting light weights again. Two years later, he was stronger than he had ever been before in his life, deadlifting over 300 pounds. If his friends needed help moving furniture, it would not be a problem anymore.

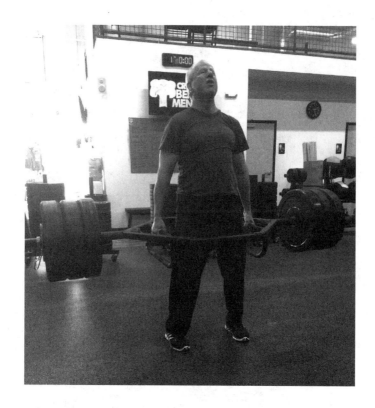

Figure 7.2. At 66, Steven is stronger than ever.

Now others have followed Fred's StrongPath choice, each case breaking away from the Frail Trail and opening a new path. The new paths have given birth to new visions of the future that support much different, stronger, and far more positive internal self-images. This is where everyone must start to establish the necessary mental foundation upon which to build a new physical reality and live a new path filled with all of the thrills and stimulating choices that greatly increased strength and health will open for them.

In our next case study, we'll get to see in more detail Steven's choice to follow the StrongPath and how he was able to continue to improve in strength, despite the medical setbacks he experienced.

CASE STUDY: STEVEN

We wanted to conduct our own tests so that you'd be able to relate to regular people and see the improvements they have experienced in a short period of time. Fred's been doing resistance training for decades and is still constantly setting personal records. His strength and health at 85 make him an "outlier" now, and there are probably no 85-year-olds who can become like Fred in their remaining years if they are starting from scratch. Because of this, we had Steven (age 66) act as a test case for this research, to show that if you are 60–70 and have a health history as troubled as his, you still have a shot at becoming your own version of what Fred has achieved. You already know Steven's story and how he had already bounced back from serious health setbacks and extreme weakness, but just so you can see that people can improve even when they're already working out regularly, let's take a look at Steven's trajectory.

During the first 16-week period, Cullen reported the following: Steven had been a consistent training client of personal trainer Cullen B. Weber, CSCS, prior to entering this study. He is an adult male who had experienced some relatively severe medical emergencies, requiring surgery several years prior to the beginning of his training at Canyon Fitness. He began training at Canyon with Cullen 3 days per week for several months prior to the beginning of the study program. During his previous training period, Steven made a great deal of progress in his overall strength and movement capacity, and as such, he came into the study already having achieved significant change. Steven should be considered an advanced lifter according to definitions set forth by the American College of Sports Medicine (ACSM) in the United States due to his training frequency and relative knowledge of lifting techniques.

Upon entry into the preliminary training contract, the first session was used to test Steven's strength using the standard barbell bench press, barbell squat and dead lift, and pull-up. A strength program was then used to train Steven approximately three times per week for approximately 16 weeks. Cullen, who was also the personal trainer and strength coach for this study, wrote this strength program. The program consisted of a variety of strength-training exercises that cycled through approximately every 6 weeks. Muscle groups were trained on specific days, though the same specific exercises were not always used. Rather than repetitively use the same exercises, a dynamic collection of exercises that can be classified as pushing, pulling, hip hinging, or squatting were used in organized patterns. The goal of the programming was to consistently train each muscle group without continually offering those muscle groups the same task to accomplish.

Training loads consisted of intermediate and advanced lifting protocols calling for multiple sets of each exercise performed at maximal effort for approximately 4–6 repetitions at 85 percent of 1-rep max capacity, and 8 to 12 repetitions at 65–75 percent of 1-rep max capacity.[7] He performed 4–5 sets of each assigned exercise and approximately 3–4 exercises were assigned for him to accomplish each day.

Training frequency and duration were affected during this period by personal leaves of absence and occasional Colorado weather conditions. This resulted in an extended training time in some instances.

Steven presented with a baseline bench-press strength apex of 155 pounds using the traditional barbell. After 4 months of strength training, he was able to achieve a maximal lift of 170 pounds using the same equipment. He could deadlift 255 pounds. After 16 weeks of training, he was able to achieve a dead lift of 300 pounds. Steven presented with a baseline back-squat capability of 155 pounds, and toward the end of his training, he was able to perform a 225-pound back squat. Steven began the study able to accomplish one full body-weight strict pull-up; he could achieve four strict pull-ups through full range of motion by the end of his first 4 months of training. The results in Figure 7.3 indicate his improvement by percentages relative to his original strength. Steven was able to achieve 110 percent of his bench-press strength, 145 percent of his back-squat strength, and 118 percent of his dead lift strength.

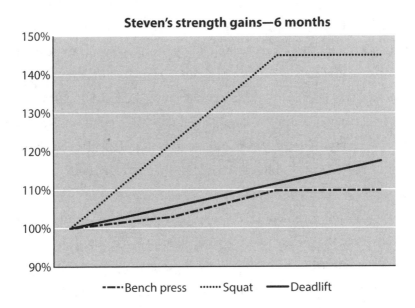

Steven's strength gains—6 months

Steven was the most advanced athlete to enter the study during this session. Cullen uses the word "athlete" here to describe any participant engaging in advanced fitness and strength activities. Steven's progression is impressive because, even though he entered the program with a strong training background, he was still able to make very positive improvements.

As one would expect with a regularly trained individual, Steven's gains were modest in terms of percentage gains relative to what a novice lifter would experience. His increases in strength are appropriate for an athlete who already has impressive strength. What we did observe during this cycle of training for Steven was an improvement in what would previously have been considered a weak area. Steven's baseline testing indicated some weaknesses in lumbopelvic hip complex flexibility and stability along with observed ankle instability. Due to this, an effort was made to especially focus on exercises that would attack those weaknesses for purposes of building strength. The result can be observed in Steven's back-squat improvement. The posterior chain (glutes, hamstrings, lats) strengthening combined with improved back-squat technique due to increased hip flexibility resulted in the most staggering improvement for his strength. This indicates that even with a history of training experience, Steven was able to achieve continued improvement in his overall ability. Even after so many of the neuromuscular adaptations had been accomplished, he was still able to achieve positive adaptations to muscle tissue, resulting in improved capacity.

Steven's improvement in his pull-up output is noteworthy, because we observed that while improvement to total force output in his previous training resulted in his ability to accomplish one body-weight pull-up, continued training with higher volume in the 65–75 percent strength sets resulted in improved strength endurance capacity.

One-Year Update

After 12 months of programmed training, Steven is still growing stronger. He has achieved increased gains to his dead lift, reaching a peak of 325 pounds. Recently he had a minor decline to 320 pounds. That was related to some back stiffness. He has continued to achieve between four and five strict body-weight pull-ups and is able now to do 5 sets with differing grips in rapid succession. When Steven began this program, his weight was approximately 190 pounds. He shed some fat through his training and at the time of the previous report was weighing in around 184 pounds. At the writing of this 12-month report, Steven has added substantial lean mass, and his weight has increased to approximately 194 pounds. Thus, for him to remain capable of producing multiple sets of 4–5 strict pull-ups in spite of his weight increasing demonstrates that both his strength and endurance in this area are improving. He also set a new personal bench-press record of 205 pounds during the week before this report.

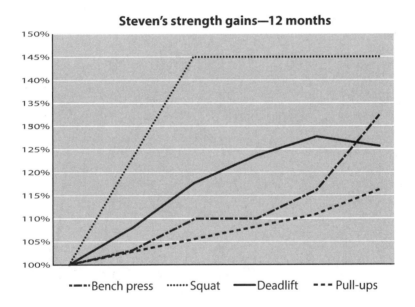

Steven's strength gains—12 months

CHAPTER 8

Making the Mental Shift to the StrongPath

LET'S STEP BACK into the world we all live in and examine in more detail the forces dragging us farther along the Frail Trail that is the default path for most of us today. As time goes by, we become less active because of the nature of the modern world. As we age, technology advances too and more services become available to us. Online shopping is starting to eclipse all the commerce in brick-and-mortar stores, so there is less of a need to walk through a mall anymore. Instead, click a few buttons and things will be brought to your door. Customer service keeps getting better with someone to carry your grocery bags if you like, and an electric scooter awaits us in Walmart in case we have trouble walking the aisles.

We start to accept our physical decline as a natural part of life. This simple expectation makes it all too easy to relax into dependence and frailty. We see it as good and right that so many "conveniences" are all around. The problem is that the process accelerates the downward spiral, making us much weaker and sicker than we otherwise would be. It literally wastes our bodies and makes us much less capable than we could be if we didn't have so much to lean on. It's great to have assistance as backup, but sadly those crutches have become the default way of life. As a result, they've become expected and we rely heavily on them.

It's easy to see how and why we slip, largely unconsciously, into a self-image guided by conventional wisdom and reinforced by our evolving modern environment. As we embrace the general expectation of growing weakness with age and envision future further decline in our imagination, we decline unnecessarily.

We now know what the looming choice is and what the overwhelming advantages are. Now we will turn to the practical mechanics of making the choice and turning that choice into a habit.

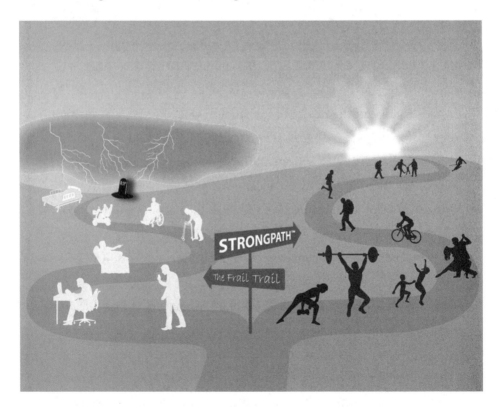

Figure 8.1. The StrongPath vs. The Frail Trail

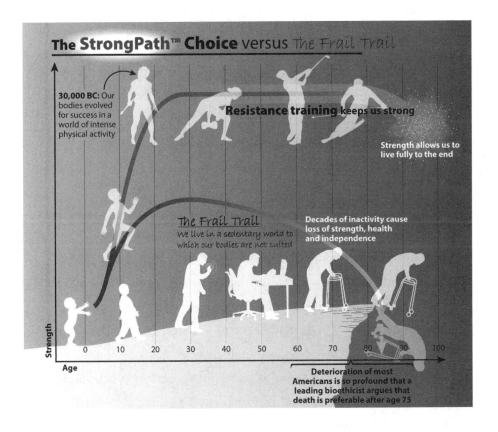

The StrongPath™ **Choice** versus The Frail Trail

30,000 BC: Our bodies evolved for success in a world of intense physical activity

Resistance training keeps us strong

Strength allows us to live fully to the end

The Frail Trail
We live in a sedentary world to which our bodies are not suited

Decades of inactivity cause loss of strength, health and independence

Strength

Age

Deterioration of most Americans is so profound that a leading bioethicist argues that death is preferable after age 75

When an image of the future has become a habit of thought, it becomes part of our unconscious, something affecting the way we automatically see things without analysis. It becomes the unspoken presumption. Its influence precedes conscious thought arising in our mind before we can consciously think.

Therefore, it is not readily changed by simply "wanting" to change it. A slower mental aspect of awareness, in this case conscious thought, regardless of how intelligent, is not directly able to lead or manage impulses seated in older, simpler, and faster parts of our nervous system that launch before we can think.

> When an image of the future has become a habit of thought, it becomes part of our unconscious, something affecting the way we automatically see things without analysis.

Habits, therefore, persist with a stubbornness that must be acknowledged and addressed. The way we change an unconscious habit of thought, like self-image, is to use the same process that formed the habit initially: Focus on a new image. Look at Figure 8.1. It is an image of two possible futures, leading to entirely different qualities of life. Which path will you take?

Change Your Mental Habits

Habits are born of repetition. Visit Figure 8.1 often. Make a decision about which path you will choose and begin to see yourself on it. This book is planting the seeds of this new vision of what your future holds in terms of strength, vigor, and health as you age. This book is talking about real life, not theory, about things that people like you are doing. Things that you can do, too. In the case studies that you read, you will learn about members in our test group and how they got started and have progressed. Each case will teach you how different people at different ages and in different health circumstances joined the StrongPath and how they have succeeded. You will see how it has been done in simple, practical terms.

Our website, Strongpath.com, will help flood your awareness with continuously updated science. On our site, you can read about others from all walks of life and their real-life success. And you will be able to post yours, too. We also will have first-class strength coaches available online to answer questions and give advice.

Objectively tracking your growing strength as your capacity to work out steadily increases will keep your motivation strong. Recording observations about feeling stronger and reclaiming abilities you thought were behind you are things you will enjoy recounting to others. Looking in the mirror and seeing an improving image will have a profound impact. Repeating these simple actions over a short period of time will radically change your self-image for the better and brighten your vision of what your future looks like. Repetition will automatically replace old habits with new ones. Your new self-image will become so central to your life that you will, by habit, do whatever it takes to defend it and prevent inroads.

BEWARE OF NEGATIVE THOUGHT PATTERNS

The opposite, a downward mental spiral, can happen as well and is equally powerful in its effects. We want to review that process too, so that you will be more aware of it when it occurs and be more alert to the danger.

How does the body influence the mind? If we are feeling strong and healthy, it is easy to have a positive attitude about life. On the other hand, if we are in pain, our thoughts and feelings darken. Let's assume that your lower back is in pain. You of course start to move more cautiously—not bending too much, avoiding lifting things—favoring that back. You become a person with a "bad back"—in your mind at least. Being a person with a "bad back," you stop lifting large, then medium, then small things, even when you are not in pain. You stop carrying grocery bags. The result is a progressive physical decline, an accelerating downward spiral, brought on by inactivity, a change in behavior inspired by pain and cemented by a self-image that now includes being a person with a "bad back."

So what do you do if your back hurts so much you don't want to pick up those grocery bags? How do you keep from falling into a destructive downward spiral? You begin with one key fact about your body: Your muscles will rise to a challenge and get remarkably stronger at any point, well into very old age, if you incrementally begin to address a weakness. You can depend on this.

When you're happy you smile, but not always necessarily in that sequence. Internal happiness will indeed bring a smile to someone's face. But have you noticed that if you are unhappy and you simply smile, the feeling of happiness still rises internally as a result of the physical action of smiling?[1] That important observation demonstrates that the body does influence and shape the mind as readily as the mind can influence and shape the body.

> Your muscles will rise to a challenge and get remarkably stronger at any point, well into very old age, if you incrementally begin to address a weakness.

Steven has experienced firsthand how profoundly changing his body profoundly changed his mind and he has also seen it in others. Korby is a man in his late 60s who was born and raised a short walk from the beach. All his life he loved to surf. A few years ago, he was despairing and ready to give up surfing, because he was suffering from increased back and shoulder pain. He also was starting to lose the ability to lift his arms over his head and several of his fingers were becoming increasingly numb. When Korby approached Steven, Steven suggested that he start coming to the gym with him.

At first Korby tired quickly on the elliptical machine, but soon he was zipping along and covering several miles at a quick pace. Soon after, he began strength training with light weights. Not only did Korby's strength increase rapidly, but the numbness also left his fingers. His shoulders strengthened, and with gradual stretching, Korby discovered that his flexibility returned. As his core got stronger, his back pain began to disappear. After only a year, he was heading back out into the waves with gusto once again. Confronted with the fork in the road, Korby abandoned the Frail Trail and took the StrongPath. This one decision changed his entire life: The surfboard, the sun, the sparkling sea in the morning, and a big smile were his once again. And to think he almost gave it all up.

Like Korby, you need to learn how to safely work your muscles. Don't wait until you are falling apart in some way before learning how to strengthen your body in a balanced, symmetrical way. If you already have a bad back, for example, it's not just your back muscles that are letting you down. Your core muscles in the front are weak, too, and those need to be strengthened so you can regain the balance in your physical system.

As you do the work to strengthen your whole system, it becomes more upright. Your skeleton becomes realigned. All of this is possible. There is virtually no "bad" body part that will not improve with careful work and rehabilitation, unless a condition has proceeded to the point where the bones are actually degraded. At that point, it is no longer just a muscle and tissue issue. As long as we're dealing with weak muscles, an intelligently pursued exercise program that starts from the point of "let's work to strengthen it" can make huge changes.

What is your plan of action when you're feeling pain? We recommend the following:

- Gather information.

- Seek professional advice from a physical therapist or a qualified exercise physiologist. The American College of Sports Medicine and the National Strength and Conditioning Association have websites that will help you find a qualified trainer in your area.

- Be willing to listen and work on what ails you.

- Address the issues: Rehab the back; work on the shoulder. Reject the pain and weakness you begin with as an outcome, and be ready to transform the situation. You can grow strong again and resume physical activity once you have tackled your ailment.

- Over the long term, you need to make your body strong enough to support your entire system. In other words, you need to get on and stay on the StrongPath.

The truth is, within 2 or 3 months, most issues will improve significantly enough that you will become confident that it's possible to change the entire trajectory of decline into one of improvement.

Fact

Muscles naturally weaken with age—starting as early as age 30—so you need to keep working them to retain strength and power. The good news is that your investment in exercise can yield quick returns. Studies have found that just 10 weeks of weight workouts can dramatically improve strength, power, mobility, and agility, even in men and women in their 70s and 80s.[2]

Once you experience improvement in one area, you will start to become eager about making more progress. Your thoughts will shift to *What can I tackle next?* You will become psychologically ready to tackle challenges in many different areas of your life that once seemed to set permanent limits on what you could realistically achieve. Physical improvement sets the stage for general improvement: being the best *you* that is possible.

The key will be to tackle and achieve success in small increments, so that nothing seems too daunting or unachievable. Fundamental change in body and mind is an overwhelming challenge if approached as something that you intend to accomplish in one bite based on willpower. But you can do it, if you have a smart and simple plan of action specifically tailored to something you need to fix in your life that will really make a difference, like rehabilitating a "bad back." Do that. Have success. Learn more about your body and your muscles overall and how any of them can be made dramatically stronger. Experience the liberating results of a focused effort. Then go on to another challenge and begin living a life of getting stronger and more capable as you age. For example, Fred is still doing this. He is currently working at becoming a faster, stronger skier than he has ever been before in his entire life.

> The truth is, within 2 or 3 months, most issues will improve significantly enough that you will become confident that it's possible to change the entire trajectory of decline into one of improvement.

A Mental Exercise: Attention

Let's take a moment and get comfortable with introspection. It is an important skill. Your attention is the master control lever of your awareness. Attention places mind, and its focus determines your experience. In fact, you are only aware of the things that receive your attention, and you are largely in control. Watch and monitor what your attention is doing. You will be surprised to find that habit is largely consuming this most precious resource. You have probably been oblivious to this because habits are preformed virtually unconsciously, until you make it a point to pay them attention and consciously observe them.

Instead of allowing habit to dictate where you spend your attention, learn to become an objective observer of it. This is an essential skill that

> Instead of allowing habit to dictate where you spend your attention, learn to become an objective observer of it.

will place a life-changing transformation within your reach. Think of it as creating a new awareness inside you, a new self that is part of you but has an independent perspective of its own.

Try this: Take a moment right now. Begin by shifting your focus inward. Become aware of the thoughts and impulses flooding your mind, especially those that repeat themselves so insistently that they seem to be running on automatic. For now, don't try to do anything about them. Simply create a mental space between you and them and watch. Simply observing your critical thoughts without judging them is a more effective way to tame them than pressuring yourself to change or denying their validity.[3]

What does this mean, exactly? It seems reasonable to assume that everything going on inside your head is *you*. In other words, the swirling thoughts are inherently a part of you. That is a misconception. It would be as if your immune system blithely assumed that everything within your skin was an essential part of yourself, not to be challenged. We know that immune systems don't behave that way, and in fact recognize unwanted intruders for what they are. This is what you must develop as an inner observer.

When you first look inside, what you see is not important. What's important is to begin to recognize that the many things going on in your head are not an essential part of you. That means that the urges that come and go, the repetitive trains of thought, advertisement jingles, habitual worries, and everyday anxieties are separate from *you*. They are largely habitual inner forces competing for your attention, and it is your decision to grant them that attention or not. The goal is to develop the conscious ability to do just that.

A perfect example is anger. If you are a successful inner observer and you notice an angry urge arising, something interesting follows: You won't accept ownership. Instead, you will be able to simply note that anger has emerged, or called for your attention. As an objective observer, you will know that you have the choice of attending to it and indulging the feeling by allowing it to manifest in your words and deeds or not. Suddenly, this simple shift in your attention places you in the driver's seat, not stuck as a passenger along for a ride determined by unconscious habit.

We use the phrase "attention commerce" to describe what is going on inside our minds. Your attention is the pot of gold, the currency that your inner potentials can use to purchase their existence and opportunities. They can be creative or destructive, beneficial or harmful, but they are always longing to be expressed and anxious that we attend to them. Observe and feel the inner tension. Notice that when you focus your attention on one thing it looms large, and other things fall away in importance. Your choice of focus changes your internal feeling and emotions.

With practice, you will learn to complete this exercise in a detached and objective manner. Your ability to develop a clear-eyed view of the competition for your attention will be a breakthrough moment. Down the road, this skill will be critical to controlling your powers of attention—making deliberate choices rather than letting haphazardly collected old habits rule. This ability will help you notice and avoid self-inflicted stress and open subconscious pathways of change.

Where can you turn your attention so that it is inherently away from the worry and anxiety that produces harmful stress? The present moment. This is your true refuge from mental stress. Actual stressful situations may exist in the present moment, requiring action, but mentally generated stress does not exist there. This is true, because thinking is a slow and complex function that takes processing time. It lags the present moment by half a second or more. To become absorbed in the raw sensory input is to be separated in time from the cognitive universe where worry exists. That can happen, because we experience sensations much faster than we can think about things. These are simple facts that reflect the biological mechanics of our nervous system, but their implications and impacts are extraordinary. They relate directly to the practice of mindfulness, which refers to the mental state of being focused in the present moment. This practice first emerged around 1500 BC and has had a profound impact on the development of Taoism, Buddhism, Sufism, and mystic Christian and Jewish practices. Tai chi and kung fu employ mindfulness. This ancient practice brought focused breath awareness to many Westerners as an integral component of physical training,[4] yielding superlative results. Today, mindfulness is used in clinical psychology to treat anxiety, depression, and pain.

Stress

Good stress is the kind that motivates us to take action. The fight-or-flight response makes our bodies physically ready to fight or flee. It is important when a real-life situation inspires the response, and it might even save our lives. Once we act, the situation soon ends, and we naturally cycle into a regenerative phase. Bad stress is mental anxiety, worry. It triggers our fight-or-flight chemistry too, but it can go on without end, never allowing the body to properly regenerate. This erodes our physical health and can shorten our lives.

There is a better grasp of mind-body connections in scientific terms. Elizabeth Stanley, PhD, served as a US Army intelligence officer during the 1990s. She began practicing mindfulness to deal with stress of deployment theaters like those in Bosnia and Macedonia. This led to her creation of a training program for those that had prolonged exposure to high-stress environments. To better inoculate soldiers to stress before deployment stress, Dr. Stanley developed MMFT—Mindfulness-Based Mind Fitness Training.[5]

She looked at the challenge, combining what she had learned from her military experience and mindfulness training with scientific research expertise. She found serious scientific partners in 2007 and was approached by funding organizations. In 2008, they put together a study with forty-seven Marine reservists who were preparing for combat deployment to Iraq. Thirty of the group received 8 weeks of MMFT, and seventeen did not. The results from those who received the training were better than expected. This triggered two more studies of troops deploying to Afghanistan and another embedded into the United States Marine Corps School of Infantry. "MMFT became the first mindfulness-based training program to have its beneficial effects with military populations documented in peer-reviewed scientific journals."[6]

Leaving service with the rank of captain, Dr. Stanley is an associate professor at Georgetown and founder of the Mind Fitness Training Institute.

A focus of attention inherently allows us to leave behind internally generated anxiety and worry. This shift of attention is accomplished by focusing on physical sensations, which inherently occur in the present moment. Stanley explains that when attention is focused on body sensation, you give a workout to the part of your brain that is the primary player in self-regulating stress. This focus also gives the brain reassurance based on real-time observations, communicating in effect "all clear"—the body is stable and OK at the moment.[7]

Dr. Stanley's research partners also have studied the brain's response to stress in average citizens, elite athletes, and members of military

Special Forces. According to the report on inoxygenmag.com, they found that elite performers were better at staying calm in the face of stress after 8 weeks of mindfulness training; nonelite performers began to resemble the elite. When faced with stress, those who had received the training maintained their center, which was verified by calmer heart rates and slowed breathing. Dr. Stanley and her colleagues made another key discovery: Immediately after a workout, our brains are better able to build neurons and establish the rewiring that helps us handle stress.[8] Applying this insight and integrating key aspects of mindfulness can importantly advance the development of StrongPath training.

> **Immediately after a workout, our brains are better able to build neurons and establish the rewiring that helps us handle stress.**

When developing his Transformational Psychology course in attention mechanics, Steven became aware of Dr. Stanley and her work through retired lieutenant colonel Dave Grossman, a graduate of Ranger School who later became a professor of psychology at West Point. Grossman's first book, *On Killing: The Psychological Cost of Learning to Kill in War and Society*, includes a compelling analysis of the ultra-high stress physiological processes involved with killing another human being. Since retiring from the Army, he has founded a research group and educates law enforcement officers and soldiers on how to achieve better outcomes when faced with potentially lethal encounters. He also speaks to civilian groups and teaches them how to deal with the aftermath of violent events, like school shootings.

We now have a growing body of new understanding built on scientific investigation that shows us how to better handle our stress. These techniques can be applied by everyone. In the case study that follows, we will learn how a petite homemaker increases her strength and self-image by choosing the StrongPath.

CASE STUDY: MARY

Mary is a 58-year-old homemaker. She is petite and thin. This test wasn't her first time to the gym: Mary spent the decade before the strength test working out. In fact, she had been hitting the gym 5 days a week for many years.

When Mary began the study, she could pull up approximately 80 pounds of her weight, and by the end of her training, she was able to achieve a full 98-pound body-weight pull-up. The results in Figure 8.3 display her improvement in percentages relative to her original strength. Respectively, Mary was able to achieve 117 percent of her bench-press strength, 105 percent of her front squat strength, 157 percent of her dead lift strength, and 121 percent of her pull-up strength.

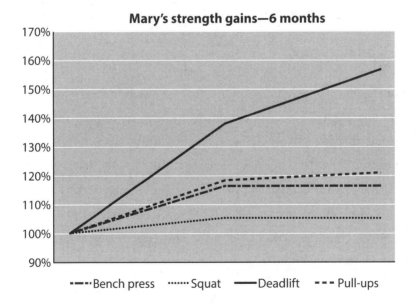

Fear Factor

The gym never really scared Mary. Her only hesitation on certain days was the unknown: What was Cullen going to throw her way during a training session? What was in store for her when she arrived at the gym? And while nutrition wasn't a fear factor for Mary, it continues to be the most challenging part of her fitness and overall health regime. She has to work on watching what she eats regularly. It's hard to fight the cravings. As for the gym? She's got that down.

Biggest Surprise

Since Mary already worked out regularly, she felt she was on top of her health. However, by being pushed to lift heavier weight, she suddenly discovered not only could she do more but that at 58, she was also in the best shape of her life.

Benefits

While leaner and able to see more muscle definition, Mary got a boost in an unexpected way: Her self-image was enhanced, because she was able measure her success by her increased lifting. Mary has fibromyalgia as well as adrenal and thyroid issues. She's found that her years of exercise help her combat the fatigue and pain brought on by the Minnesota humidity before she moved to Denver. She said that despite an excessively humid summer recently, the program seems to have helped diminish those symptoms.

Words of Wisdom

"Just get to the gym," said Mary. Once you're there, and you start moving, you'll be able to increase what you're doing. If you can swing it, Mary suggests using a trainer to guide you, because a trainer will push you to work harder than you might push yourself. Mary believes if you're strong and healthy, you'll live longer and be happier.

A month or two after the test period, Mary told Steven with a big smile that she and her husband Peter had found a wonderful, large china hutch in a small shop. Once they purchased it, the staff told them that they didn't have anyone who could help them load it into the truck. Mary said she was prepared to jump into action and load the furniture with her husband. Mary had just recently set new personal records in deadlifting, which is exactly the kind of exercise that translates into the ability to safely lift heavy items. She said she tested herself and found she had no problem lifting one end of the piece. The staff eventually did help them load it, but once home, Mary and Peter took over on their own, lifting and unloading the hutch by themselves without any additional manpower. She said to Peter, "We can do this," and off Peter and little 98-pound Mary went!

Experiences like this powerfully reorient self-image. Breaking free from the presumption that age and time are inexorably overpowering our physical abilities is an essential shift in self-knowledge that opens up horizons we mistakenly thought we'd never see.

Mind Games: Steven's Solution

The CDC confirms Mary's experience and states, "Strength training, particularly in conjunction with regular aerobic exercise, can also have a profound impact on a person's mental and emotional health. . . . Strength

Continued

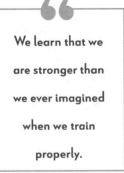

> We learn that we are stronger than we ever imagined when we train properly.

training provides similar improvements in depression as those achieved with anti-depressant medications."[9]

The immune response, and even the psychological shift, is system-wide, complex, and profound. Added to this are the psychologically uplifting effects of self-discovery that lead to much-improved self-knowledge. We learn that we are stronger than we ever imagined when we train properly.

One-Year Update

After 12 months of training, Mary continues to get stronger. She can now deadlift 170 pounds. She can also do five full-range-of-motion, palms-forward pull-ups and bench-press 95 pounds.

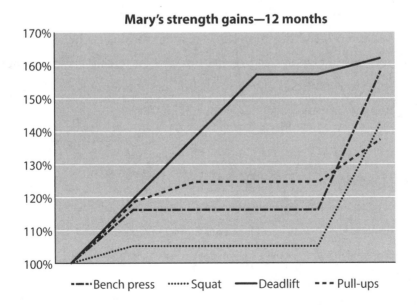

Mary's strength gains—12 months

CHAPTER 9

Habit, Willpower, and Our Ancient Brains

THERE ARE THREE automatic forces that are at work on all of us: attitude, physical habits, and beliefs. When it comes to choosing the StrongPath and beginning an exercise program, it's helpful to understand the ways they can affect our success. The attitude you currently hold about your physical body or the value of strength training may have become reinforced by your habits and resistance to the new information that could benefit your health. Attitude is often an emotional response and can be a powerful force you may need to consciously reject. The repetition of habit is what can help keep you on the Strong-Path, but it's also what can derail you if your bad habits are already ingrained. But as we've discussed, we can't leave this up to willpower. To be successful in battling sarcopenia, you must make strength and cardio training of adequate intensity a habit versus a conscious choice, and we'll show you how to establish this habit so it lasts. Tied into all of this are our beliefs, which are essentially mental habits or how we think about things like aging. If you have long believed that you are doomed to the Frail Trail, then you will fail. Knowing more about how attitude, habits, and beliefs affect our brains is critical to your ability to remain mentally motivated on your physical transformation.

Attitude

To get off the default life path that currently has you on the road to sarcopenia and all of its consequences will require some serious attitude shifts. Even if you are ambivalent, beware. You will still need to shift your attitude. Research on social influence indicates that when we are unsure, we are likely to adjust our judgments in favor of the group standard. There is a rational desire and an emotional urge to take into account the presumed knowledge of others. This is perilous when a group is largely misinformed or uninformed on a matter, because it can cause people to adopt an observable trend as conclusive and make decisions accordingly with very little real information leading the way. This is the case with knowledge about sarcopenia and its cure today. And the downward slope we are on is psychologically slippery precisely because it is so easy to accept.

How we feel about someone, something, or some topic can easily influence us more strongly and move us in a deeper way than we objectively know.

One problem is that you currently have attitudes and feelings about what your body can and cannot—or perhaps should not—do physically. Such attitudes likely originated with a negative personal health episode and were perhaps reinforced over time by further episodes. That was certainly Steven's experience. His lower back went out one day when he turned as he lifted his desk. It left him bent over and in great pain. This was followed by a few more episodes where his back went out again doing much less challenging activities. Soon, he developed an attitude about being asked to lift or move things. He began to reflexively decline requests to help others, out of fear of aggravating his back. The more automatic the decision became, the more powerful the link was between his attitude and the decision. Going forward, this meant that he was more likely to use his attitude alone as a source of knowledge regarding decision-making in related circumstances. The more often he did this, the more resistant he became to new information. This downward spiral makes attitudes, particularly strong negative attitudes, difficult to change by new information alone.

For the moment, think of attitude as a habitual emotional response and shortcut to decision-making. The special force of attitude is emotion. How we feel about someone, something, or some topic can easily influence us more strongly and move us in a deeper way than we objectively know. Interestingly, given our subject matter, studies demonstrate that the intensity of implicit attitudes may be measured by gauging muscle tension while a person is thinking about an attitude object.[1]

Another form of measurement for whether something is an unconscious attitude as opposed to a conscious thought is the speed at which people react to an attitude object.[2] Both of these are keys to understanding the power of attitude.

Self-conscious awareness arises rather slowly, taking a half second or more. An emotional response to something can occur much more quickly, change our blood chemistry, rev up our fight-or-flight response, and make our muscles tense and ready to act. In other words, this is an example of emotions occurring ahead of conscious awareness and therefore having the advantage of setting the mental and physiological context of thought. Little wonder it is so difficult for words of reason to move us when something has triggered a flash of anger, fear, loathing, or conversely, smitten adoration.

Exercise: Attitude

Mentally picture an actor or a politician that you do not like. Look inside and notice that your feeling about this person—your attitude—arises faster than you can think. With thought, you can reexamine the reasons for your dislike, but for the moment, just notice that your feelings, your emotional reaction to his or her image, comes first; this is often enough to cause you to quickly decide not to see his or her new movie or not to vote for him or her, if someone suggests that you do so, without further consideration. This is how attitude can act as a default basis for decision. Attitudes are useful, because they are a very efficient, nearly effortless way of determining positions and courses of action. In many cases, it works well to be quick and consistent in the way we judge and handle things, but not always.

Attitudes will determine the course of your thoughts and actions unless you override them in favor of adopting another path of thought and action when appropriate. And you can.

Physical Habits

There are good and bad physical habits. Habits are the behaviors that we have repeated so often that they now launch automatically, unconsciously, whenever they are triggered. They may be triggered by time of day, place, a thought or mood, an associated activity, or a repeating circumstance. For example, brushing your teeth is likely a good habit that is part of your morning routine on a daily basis without conscious consideration.

Think how burdensome and time-consuming brushing your teeth

would be if every morning you consciously had to decide to brush your teeth. *Should I brush my teeth again today? Is it really worth the effort? Would it matter if I just skipped today? It's the weekend and I don't plan to go out. But, maybe someone will come by and I don't want to have bad breath* . . . Just dithering about the decision would become a form of suffering itself and the time wasted quickly would become a substantial problem. A good habit relieves us of all this, and this is the blessing of having a brain that can and will transfer the initiation and execution of a repeated activity to a portion of our brain that need not involve the conscious attention of our mind.

The raw power of habit lies in ongoing repetition and that power is enormous. Consciously, we may have the willpower to do something once, twice, ten times. But each time, it requires a mental effort to do so, and sooner or later we tire of the effort. But a habit will launch and repeat an effort without the drag of mental effort and has the cumulative effect of something done a thousand times, ten thousand times, and more. Herman Melville marveled at its power, saying, "Yet, habit—strange thing! What cannot habit accomplish?"[3] But of course, as wonderfully beneficial as this is for a good habit, it is equally and horribly destructive for a bad habit.

> Your ability to change your life course and reach a whole new level of physical and mental ability cannot depend on conscious choice. It will only come because of training your unconscious.

You very much need and want the power of habit working for you to defeat sarcopenia. Your ability to change your life course and reach a whole new level of physical and mental ability cannot depend on conscious choice. It will only come because of training your unconscious.

James's Observations

William James made some useful observations in 1890. For example, he advised us to "make our nervous system our ally instead of our enemy" and to "make automatic and habitual, as early as possible, as many useful actions as we can"[4] while we guard against adopting bad habits by treating them like the plague they are. He saw that the more of the details of our daily life we can hand over to effortless automatic habit, the more our mind is set free to focus on its work. He also observed that no one is a more miserable than a human being who tries to use his mind for what should be the work of habit. Deliberating each day on when to go to bed or wake up, whether to exercise or not, what to eat or not eat rather than making decisions and then working on building good habits accordingly is a life of ongoing suffering and ongoing failure. James said if you are not already coasting along on mostly good habits, then your first and most urgent job is to start working on doing so.

In short, the key to success is making strength training as habitual and essential to your life as breathing. Before the habit becomes ingrained, you will be tempted to come up with excuses to avoid it. This is precisely what William James was warning us about. It leads to failure and suffering. Strength training is a critically important part of your life. It is more important than any activity or, worse still, inactivity that you might allow to push your workout aside in a weak moment. Habit alone has the continuing power to keep you strong and help make you the best you can be.

ESTABLISH A HABIT

If you're going to be exercising at home, it may begin as small as doing one push-up or one squat. More important than the size of the effort to begin with is learning how to condition a habit by trying something like the following:

- Fix the time when you're going to automatically do your push-up or squat, without thinking. Perhaps when you first wake up. Do it every day. Repetition is key to making something a habit and doing something easy, automatically every day will make the action a habit more quickly. Focus first and foremost on showing up for the routine and establishing the habit.

- Repeat the action consistently. Increase the number of repetitions incrementally every week on the same day. This will prepare you for the strength training that lies ahead.

How long does it take to form a habit? Curiously, a very seductive bad habit, such as quitting your workouts, might be established by a single episode. Michael Jordan said, "If you quit once, it becomes a habit. Never quit!" Good habits most often take longer. There is some conventional wisdom that began with the personal observations of Dr. Maxwell Maltz, a plastic surgeon in the 1950s, who observed that most patients quickly experienced a rise in self-esteem and confidence, usually within 21 days of corrective surgery. The 21-day figure became a commonly held idea on the time it takes for habit formation. But it was not backed up by real research. A scientific study in 2009 was designed to investigate the process of habit formation. Ninety-six volunteers were tested, and the time it took participants to make a chosen behavior a habit ranged from 18 to 254 days. The average was 66 days. They also noted that missing a single instance when the time came to perform the behavior did not affect the habit-formation process. But a habit did form more quickly if the behavior was routinely put in a consistent context.[5]

Establish any level of habit, then build on it. Once something becomes a habit, an automatically initiated action is in place. You will then have the platform psychologically established, and you will be building your repertoire of rote behaviors in subconscious portions of your nervous system that can be easily expanded in duration. The hard part, the part where you can stumble and fail, is in getting the effort launched before you talk yourself out of it. So, the small success of determining a time and place where you will automatically launch into a routine behavior is key. Once you establish one habit, you can add another, until a full-blown program is built that will be your vehicle for real change.

If you are going to start going to a gym, and we strongly recommend that you do, fix the days of the week and time you will be going. Do not leave the question of where or when open. This is essential. This is part of building a successful habit. If you can afford a trainer, it is a great help in many ways. I find it is easier to get myself to an appointment when I have made a commitment to someone else. This technique may help you get over the hump of establishing a habit, and the trainer will tell you what to do, so that you don't have to think about that. Less thinking helps in habit formation. So does a present-moment focus on the sensations you are experiencing during a workout.

Beliefs

Think of a belief as a habit of thought. Since belief is a relationship with information, when new and better information comes along, it is time to update a habit of thought. For example, if we mistakenly believe the decline of sedentary living is actually an unchangeable, inevitable consequence of aging, it can profoundly affect our behavior. We won't try to build muscle after a certain point, because we think that older people don't have muscle, can't have muscle, or maybe even *shouldn't* have muscle. As long as such beliefs hold sway, you will find yourself on the inevitable road to sarcopenia. Modern medicine is struggling to update its relationship with the scope and sweep of this new information, too.

Information Isn't Enough

Knowing all this isn't going to change your life. Information alone is not sufficient, and, sadly, that is why many books are read, yet few lives are changed substantially enough to set an individual on a significantly better life course. Attitude and physical habits must be adjusted, too.

It's easier to change a physical habit by developing a new routine that takes the time and place of the old habit, and, over time, we find that experiencing the uplifting benefits of successful physical improvement then reinforces the routine. This is how we can change poor physical habits by incrementally adopting new physical routines that, with repetition, become new habits.

If a negative attitude is adopted from a negative emotional experience, an efficient way to change this negative attitude is to introduce a positive emotional experience to counteract it. No amount of information will equal in emotional impact the joy of regaining a treasured physical ability you thought you had lost or perhaps attaining some thrilling new abilities that you've never had before in your life. Many such experiences have been ours, and, I promise you, they will also be yours by adopting good strength-building routines. The ongoing dramatic experience of the process will automatically shift your current attitudes and self-image. A newly forming and far abler body will bring with it a new conscious and unconscious state of mind as it develops.

Final Notes on Willpower

Our awareness is flexible and open to making new kinds of decisions and exploration, and being plastic in that sense means that you cannot wisely give it the responsibility of a rote behavior. People who have an image of themselves that says, "I'm a person of strong willpower, and willpower is the core of my success" are wrong.

That's just not the case. The core of anyone's success, bull-headed or otherwise, stems largely from habits and attitudes. Willpower should never be given a job that requires a continuing rote response, like getting yourself to the gym three times a week.

If you're serious about maintaining a particular activity, willpower has to be used only to prime the pump, to start the process, to engage in an activity with enough repetition so that it begins to be seeded in the primitive portions of your brain, down in your basal ganglia. Once it takes over launching the activity, willpower is no longer needed. There is no longer any conscious decision-making about whether or not you will go to the gym today. If it's Wednesday and it's 9:00 a.m. and that's your time, you simply go.

Fact

According to Professor Baba Shiv at Stanford University, willpower is so weak, and the prefrontal cortex is so overtaxed, that all it takes is five extra bits of information before the brain starts to give in to temptation.[6]

It's important that you don't think about whether or not to exercise. It's important because every time you open up the question to a process of decision-making consciously, you hand off the responsibility from your strong rote ability to your forever flexible chattering mind—and you will falter. It's like this: *Will I go to the gym today? Well, let's see. How do I feel? Do I really need to? I did great yesterday. I am tired. I have an important meeting.*

Face it, you'll talk yourself out of going. That's what the conscious mind loves to do. It is important that instead you begin with the intention of building a habit and not of engaging in any further decision-making. It's also important that you don't think about whether or not to exercise. It's important that you don't think about it, because every time you open it up to a process of decision-making consciously, you will falter, because conscious decision-making is *made to be flexible.*

Setting the Habit Is Key

Dr. Kaminsky runs a health and well-being center at Ball State University. He lets participants know that his research shows there is no harm in exercising when they have a cold. Instead, what is risky is taking more than a little time off when trying to establish an exercise routine because of a cold. That can lead to "falling away from the program entirely."[7]

THE LONG GAME

Boot camps and crash diets don't work, because while you may have enough willpower to show up and go through with them, let's face it, they are designed to be short. They are intended to be the opposite of habit, designed to fit your limited willpower, rather than to address your honest to goodness lifelong health needs. That's their appeal. But there's no quick fix. Retraining your mind with new habits is the only way to establish long-term change.

Old structures in your nervous system have the ability to react, to respond appropriately, in hundredths or tenths of a second faster than you can think.[8] That's why you can catch your balance before you fall over. That sophisticated action needs to be done just right and with the right amount of force and counterforce to regain your balance. It's a difficult movement to perform, and the portion of your nervous system that can do it is subconscious. This means it steps up when it needs to and acts before conscious awareness is cognizant of the situation.

Such ancient aspects of our neural and physical capability are there because they were critical to survival long before our brains developed the facility for self-conscious awareness, and they still work in the same way and at the same speed as they always have.[9] Therefore, it is helpful to have a self-image based on a better acquaintance with our physical nature. Recognizing that willpower is fleeting but that habit can repattern your nervous system will enable you to approach your exercise program with the right tools for success.

NEW, STRONGER MOTIVATION

Life experience has a complexity and special power that intellectual analysis and discussion simply do not have.

This is what will happen to you as you start to make progress with your resistance training. You will have feelings of euphoria, produced by body chemistry, when you challenge your previous personal best resistance-training record and succeed. Your source of motivation to do so again will no longer primarily come from pushing yourself with inner encouragements. Rather, you will be eager to step up, cross a personal frontier, and feel the euphoria anew. You will enjoy returning to the memories and feeling in your memory and in the sharing and retelling.

When you experience this yourself, you have knowledge that is complete. That comes with all of the exhilarating feelings. Your knowing is intimate rather than distant, full and immediate rather than detached and intellectual. This quality of knowing automatically changes your self-image, because you have done something that you have never done before. Even if each step is a small increment of improvement, having accomplished something and then experiencing the feeling that went with it—the exertion, the almost not being able to do it, and then success—is an indescribably rich and wonderful feeling. As you put together three, four, five, and more of those experiences over a period of months, then years, your entire vision of self and your estimation of your ability to accomplish things will dramatically change, and so will your future.

THINK YOUNG

When we were young, we got excited about things. We got excited about having some fun, doing something different, and exploring something new. Physical activity was almost always part of new experiences. Think about the very nature of recess: running around with abandon outside. How sad that this is ever less the case for kids today.

The good news is that delight in movement is in our nature. It is primal to human beings, young and old. Yet, over time, it is easy to become more self-conscious, disengaged from activity, and less capable of physical activity. It takes an effort to get reengaged. But once you do, all of a sudden, your body responds. You get stronger. You move faster. And you feel better.

That's why the right attitude is to try to reenter that mental space and rediscover the natural process, because it's all still there in every single one of us, waiting to well up, regardless of age or fitness level. Think about it this way: Old people can still laugh at jokes, right? That sense of fun, of being caught by surprise by something silly, and then laughing about it—it's there in us. That function and ability is the spirit in which healing occurs and in which physical growth begins again.

You *can* choose the StrongPath.

Know this: There's not a person alive who can't do these things— not a single one. Everyone has the power to dramatically change their physical and mental abilities. You simply need to show up, ready to make the choice and to engage in the process. As you do so, you will draw strength from the experience that will be your own.

Success Motivates

"To me, one important factor that makes this so amazing: It is easy to see and measure success, which is so motivating! Anyone can have success if they only start! You will never question if your better life is happening—the most important aspects are clearly measurable, so there is no doubt."

—StrongPath test group participant, Wendy Poage

THE REASONS SO few choose the StrongPath are overwhelmingly mental. But that doesn't mean you have to rely on willpower. In fact, you now know that its limitations will only cause you to fail. Instead, you must make a conscious effort to reframe both your physical and mental habits through the act of repetition. The key to your success lies in your ability to make the decision to engage in strength training an automatic response that you will follow as part of a new routine. This often begins with creating a positive self-image, one that reflects your ability to be strong and capable well into your later years, because your mental attitude has a powerful effect on your physical body. This new vision will allow your new path to emerge. Once you see improvements, you'll want to work harder and tackle the next ache and pain by building more strength. If we can do it, so can you.

In the next chapter, we're going to show you how to get started by explaining some of the science behind muscle health and why strength training works. But first, we'd like you to meet Tom, who chose the StrongPath and overcame balance and mobility issues in the case study that follows.

CASE STUDY: TOM

Tom is a 68-year-old residential interior designer. He was diagnosed with HIV in 1988. Before beginning the program, Tom reviewed our research findings and learned that HIV-positive individuals needed regular cardio and resistance training to remain healthy just like everyone else. Tom was checked by his doctor and was soon cleared to begin training. His build was slender, and he began with some balance and shoulder mobility issues.

Tom joined the group of participants later in the year but executed the same program that other participants did. He presented with some unique upper-body limitations, primarily in his shoulder mobility. And his strength gains are indicative of an individual who has had no formal training in weight lifting.

Tom improved greatly in his dead lift ability, much more than in any other lift. His improvement in core strength and general spinal stability emerged in that lift. It is also worth noting that his pull-up strength improved and became much more aligned with his body weight. Further training, focused on improving mobility in his shoulder, will likely allow him to achieve an unassisted pull-up.

Tom's shoulder mobility issue also affects his ability to execute squats. He was unable for quite some time to adequately complete a front or back squat, because he could not grasp the bar with proper form. His bench press improved with shoulder mobility work and after strengthening the joint to stabilize heavier lifts. His gradual improvement is encouraging to see, as it is an indicator of improved shoulder stability and strength.

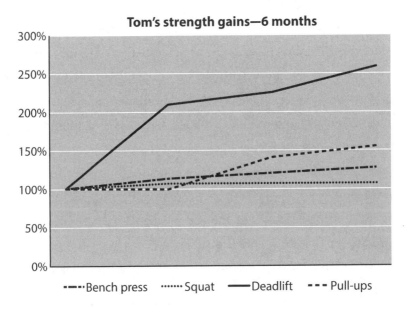

Tom's strength gains—6 months

- - · Bench press   ······· Squat   —— Deadlift   - - - Pull-ups

Fear Factor

Tom didn't know how his personal health situation might affect his ability to participate, so reading current research and frank recommendations from solid sources helped. Once his doctor cleared him, he was excited to get into a program that was specifically designed to make him stronger. Since he entered StrongPath training later than other members of our test group, he was able to meet people close to his age who were already achieving the kind of gains that he looked forward to achieving. He had some concerns about the balance and mobility issues he was having and was happy that these were assessed and taken into account as his training began.

Biggest Surprise

The biggest surprise for Tom was how quickly his strength increased. He was also surprised to experience how simple things (like turning his attention away from the gym mirrors, closing his eyes, and focusing intently on his breath, exhaling as he pushed) could suddenly make it possible to lift heavier weight. The first time Cullen had him do this, Tom was doing dumbbell bench presses. Cullen brought him 5-pound heavier dumbbells and put them in his hands and asked him to do as many reps as he could. Tom did 5 more reps than he had done with lighter weights the prior set. When Tom finished his set, Cullen praised him for doing more, and Tom said, "Yeah, but you gave me lighter weights." Tom then looked at the end of one of the weights and was amazed to see that they were heavier.

Tom learned about neuromuscular activation and that he didn't have to grow more muscle to get much stronger at first, because muscles that don't get used much don't work efficiently. Challenging them causes more existing muscle cells to join in and work, yielding more strength early on. He began to get in tune with his body's ability to shift gears, adapt, and do work by focusing and incrementally digging deeper in new ways.

Benefits

Being 68 and able to bend over and deadlift 60 pounds in the beginning and then 4 months later being able to lift 155 pounds is a radical, life-changing experience. This is not just a number. That's not what is amazing. What is incredible are all the things this means Tom can do that he could not do before. He has much more energy, ready strength, and the confidence that comes with knowing what he can do. And he is getting steadily stronger.

Words of Wisdom

"I want everyone in the HIV community, who is mentally and physically where I was at before I began, to know that if I can do it, so can you. Know that there is room for great strength gains in your life, and it can and will happen much quicker than you think. With strength will come new confidence and that will bring an overall improvement in your outlook. If you seek out a trainer, look for one who is educated in exercise physiology and is a *stickler* for good form, which is very important!"

> "I want everyone in the HIV community, who is mentally and physically where I was at before I began, to know that if I can do it, so can you."

Mind Games: Steven's Solution

After completing the initial 4 months of StrongPath training, Tom relocated out of state for professional reasons. Cullen provided Tom with follow-up training advice, and Tom looked for a good facility and a trainer to continue. He suffered an accident at home when he caught a foot in a sofa slip cover while walking through the living room and fell fast and hard on a hardwood floor, fracturing a knee cap (very hard to do), which caused a meniscus tear. He decided against surgery and opted for physical rehabilitation. Tom regained knee function and continued upper-body workouts throughout the rehab process with his knee. He realized that if he had not had the experience of working out and growing strong and learning how capable his body was of improving, he would never have had the confidence or the motivation to show up for continued strength training or to work diligently at rehab after his fall.

Continued

It was not only his body that had become much stronger; he had also become much more knowledgeable and sure of his abilities. He was no longer a person who retreated from physical activity when a problem arose. He knew about gyms and working out and immediately understood the importance of rehab disciplines after injury. He wanted to do what he could do first, rather than take to his bed and expect a doctor to fix everything. At the time of his accident, he was in a different, stronger mental and physical state than he would have been in before his Strong-Path training.

As we age, the road ahead will offer us similar challenges. Our ability to bounce back is a critical part of our future prospects. As fate had it, Tom found himself better prepared mentally and physically for an unforeseeable event, just in time.

CHAPTER 10

Getting Started: Know Your Muscles

STRONGPATH TRAINING HAS the power to shift you into an upward spiral and help you secure a far brighter future. We're dedicated to making sure you train correctly. We want you to stick with us for the long haul and stay on a healthy path. To do that, we've designed a step-by-step process based on science that includes critical, regular assessments that increase in difficulty as you progress, all with one goal in mind: a long and healthy life made up of stellar years.

We believe that a knowledge of how and why things work can help keep you on track, so in this chapter we want you to get to know your muscles. We'll explain the science behind muscle health and why it's important to train all of your muscles. We'll also give you some essential tips to keep in mind as you begin your program.

GETTING STARTED: PATTERNS OF MOVEMENT

It is human to want to emphasize our strengths and ignore our weaknesses. Most people like to exercise doing what they do best and prefer to avoid what they don't do well. Unfortunately, this type of approach to exercise will never put you on the StrongPath. It takes some humility to overcome this initial human impulse. Objective functional movement and strength assessments will determine what you need to work on. You will discover what weaknesses need special attention in your workouts to bring your strength into balance. You will begin by doing many things you don't do well and long unused muscles will struggle and complain.

Approaching exercise anew in this way will put you on a path that achieves breakthrough after breakthrough. Weaknesses that you may have imagined were permanent will be overcome and left behind. Your mind-set too will shift, and soon you will anticipate and relish the thrill of achieving still more new strengths and abilities.

How important is all of this to getting squarely on the Strong-Path? Very! Your central nervous system is command and control for movement. It learns patterns of movement. Muscles, bones, and nerves grow and strengthen in response to the movement challenges of gravity, balance, and load in real time. Or they all degrade and waste away with disuse.

If the last time you tried to get up off the floor you were 50 pounds lighter and stronger than you are now, you need to get in touch with this new reality, and you must relearn and practice safe patterns of movement. This is one of the critical lifelong things you must learn to do right and then keep doing as a habit.

Movement health equals *ability*, the opposite of which is *disability*. Movement is about much more than being adequately mechanically adapted to your world; it is an art that is fundamental to the human experience. In movement, you find the spirit, feel, and joy of life.

Our modern world is becoming movement impoverished. Kids grow up who can't skip. They never learned how. Their central nervous system has no movement pattern for it. How sad is that? At 85 years old, Fred still skips down a long hallway at his home, partly for the sheer joy of it.

THE SCIENCE OF MUSCLE HEALTH

We begin with the keystone scientific fact: Muscle health is an essential part of whole-body health. It's not just a source of strength. Muscle is an organ with multiple functions. Without strength and good muscle health, our bodies struggle to function properly. We're not here to advocate weight loss; we care about body composition, muscle mass, and strength. And about preserving the quality of your last decades of life.

In his article "The Underappreciated Role of Muscle in Health and Disease" in *The American Journal of Clinical Nutrition*, aging and longevity expert Dr. Robert R. Wolfe said, "The importance of muscle mass, strength, and metabolic function in the performance of exercise, as well as the activities of daily living (ADL), has never been questioned. Perhaps less well recognized, muscle plays a central role in whole-body protein metabolism, which is particularly important in the response to stress. Furthermore, abundant evidence points to a key role of altered muscle metabolism in the genesis, and therefore prevention, of many common pathologic conditions and chronic diseases."[1]

Part of the problem with the quest for the ideal weight is that everyone winds up focusing on the body mass index (BMI). Multiple studies have been written on the impact of obesity based on BMI, but that's pointing doctors and nutrition experts in the wrong direction, because people with a lot of muscle can have a high BMI and actually be healthier than those with lower BMIs and no muscle. Dr. Arun Karlamangla, a professor in the geriatrics division at the Geffen School, acknowledged that we should be counseling older adults on prevention: "The greater your muscle mass, the lower your risk of death."[2] That's where the focus should be.

Strength and Aging

Is a focus on strength still appropriate as we age? Yes. Strength is critical as we age. Medicine is there after a bad fall to repair injuries. But something as critical to future health as strength-based fall risk assessment is rarely performed until after the first fall occurs. Yet studies have identified the segment of the population that is at high risk for falls.[3] To date, an important opportunity for primary prevention is largely being missed. There are important prevention opportunities.

According to the Harvard Medical School special report *Strength and Power Training for Older Adults*[4]—

- Senior exercise programs tend to feature very light exercise with some stretching, but research shows that sticking with very low intensity activities is neither necessary nor especially helpful.
- Nine seniors 89-91 who participated in an 8-week strength-training study increased their strength by 174 percent.
- Even people hobbled by severe frailty or disabling arthritis, unable to do other exercises, can do strength training and benefit.
- Increased strength and endurance serves as a gateway to greater independence and participation in more pleasurable activities.
- "The full health benefits of strength and power training are available to individuals who incrementally increase the weight in their workout as they are able. As muscles strengthen and adapt they need new challenges."

The Numbers Are Clear

Our national situation is catastrophic and getting worse:

- "More than 60% of US adults do not engage in the recommended amount of activity."[5]
- "Approximately 25% of US adults are not active at all."[6]
- "Nearly half of American youth aged 12 to 21 years are not vigorously active on a regular basis."[7]
- "Participation in all types of physical activity declines strikingly as age or grade in school increases."[8]

ALL MUSCLES MATTER

StrongPath training is all about being *proactive*. A big part of having a great life is learning to dodge bullets. Before we get into the "how to" of StrongPath training principles, we want to teach you about muscle in a bit more detail, as it pertains to your soon-to-be new regime. An understanding of all of this is critical to your personal health. In later chapters, you will find detailed information explaining how you can build a lifelong program that begins from the right point for your current condition. You will discover how to integrate your workout program with your health care in a way that will yield the solid testable gains in strength and health benefits that will make both you and your doctor happy. But first you need to better understand exactly how your muscles work.

> StrongPath training is all about being *proactive*. A big part of having a great life is learning to dodge bullets.

All Your Muscles Need Exercise

There's a basic fact: Muscles that do not get exercised waste away. To maintain overall health, all major muscle groups must be adequately exercised. Doing some exercise is better than none and so it is commonly recommended, but advice like "just move more *or* walk regularly" is not all it takes to achieve and maintain strength and health. Exercising lower-body muscles by walking, for example, does not adequately exercise upper-body muscles, which will continue to waste away from disuse. A full-body exercise program is what you really need, and you can perform this in a reasonable amount of time. A great deal can be accomplished by engaging in a well-designed aerobic and strength-training program that efficiently challenges all major muscle groups during three 1-hour sessions per week.

> A great deal can be accomplished by engaging in a well-designed aerobic and strength-training program that efficiently challenges all major muscle groups during three 1-hour sessions per week.

The Whole Muscle Needs to Be Exercised

Not all muscles cells are alike. Therefore, it's important to engage in an exercise program that will adequately call upon both your slow-twitch and your fast-twitch muscle cells. This way, you exercise the entire muscle, not just a part of it.

Slow- and Fast-Twitch Muscle Cells

Slow-twitch and fast-twitch cells need to be challenged according to their natures. Slow-twitch muscle cells are designed for endurance. They are small compared to fast-twitch muscle cells. You use your slow-twitch muscles to keep your posture erect, walk or bicycle at a calm pace, wash the dishes, and other day-to-day activities during which you would rarely break a sweat. Slow-twitch muscle cells do not fire all at once. They typically fire asynchronously.[9] This allows some to work while others rest, so they act like a tag team, providing each other relief while work continues at an even pace.

Fast-twitch muscle cells are much larger than slow-twitch cells. Their job is to help you do hard things that take a lot of force in a short time, such as picking up something heavy, bounding up a flight of stairs, lifting yourself off the floor, or catching your balance when you stumble so you do not fall. You will also engage fast-twitch muscle cells when you perform high-intensity resistance training.

Fast-twitch muscles cells increasingly activate when around 75 percent or more of your capacity for strength is engaged and you still need more to do something. When they do get activated, they begin synchronously firing with sudden force. At high levels of exertion, they exhaust in around 30 seconds to 2 minutes. They are what sprinters use for a 100- or 200-yard dash. This is why sprint events are short. Depending on your genetics and habitual patterns of behavior, fast-twitch cells may be half or more of your muscle mass and a great aspect of their nature is that you can adequately exercise them in a very short period of time. You can make great gains in strength with a workout program that effectively engages them as well without the need to spend a lot of extra time in the gym.

Both kinds of muscle cells are important for long-term health. Therefore, both need exercise or they will be lost. Fast-twitch muscle cells are generally the first to be lost, because they most often suffer chronic disuse. Your exercise program must be designed to challenge both kinds of muscle cells adequately throughout your lifetime.

Proportion and Symmetry of Muscle Development Is Critical

As you prepare to embark on the StrongPath, keep the following in mind:

- Muscles work as a system.

- Any part of your body that is smaller and weaker in proportion to other parts will be subject to injury.

- From the beginning, work with the same weight on each side of your body. You will likely begin with one side being stronger than the other. Nevertheless, begin with lower-weight dumbbells that both sides can handle, for example, and do the same number of repetitions on each side. Progress by increasing weight only as both sides can handle the challenge.

- It is a serious error to get into a habitual routine that exercises the same few muscles on each occasion.

If you currently go to a gym, you probably have noticed that the treadmill and exercise bike areas are much more populated than the resistance machine area, which in turn is more populated than the free-weight area. Notice too that many people habitually go to the same few machines they frequent and do the same things. For as long as you have seen them, they have not advanced or grown stronger, and their bodies have not significantly changed over time.

Some become swimming or bicycling enthusiasts, for example, and exercise strenuously, but these activities aren't weight-bearing, so they won't improve bone mass or density. Some become marathon runners, developing endurance and slow-twitch muscle cells, but do not significantly gain muscle mass as their regimen neglects fast-twitch muscle cells and actually cannibalizes them to supply amino acids to critical body tissue during long, grueling events.

Just doing something, even something strenuous, does not make for a good lifelong StrongPath program. To stay on track, you need to challenge all your muscles and all your muscle cells and to reference your strength, body composition, and bloodwork over time to know you are on the beam toward excellent long-term health.

> Just doing something, even something strenuous, does not make for a good lifelong StrongPath program. To stay on track, you need to challenge all your muscles.

According to Harvard Medical:

"Exercise delivers powerful, wide-ranging health benefits," but to reap its full rewards you must perform several different types of activities on a regular basis. Do strength exercises for all major muscle groups (legs, hips, back, chest, abdominals, shoulders, arms) at least twice weekly.[10]

MUSCLE HEALTH IS an essential part of whole-body health, not just a source of strength. Unused muscles waste away. That's why it's so important to exercise all of them. To achieve the maximum benefit on the StrongPath, you will have to step outside of your comfort zone and the types of repetitive activities you have always done and know you are good at and instead challenge yourself to work on those areas that are weaker. You will need to establish new patterns of movement to avoid muscular atrophy and to ensure overall health and disease prevention. Understanding that all muscles matter and the difference between slow-twitch and fast-twitch muscles will help improve your ability to work out. Don't be afraid to engage those fast-twitch muscles with a varied resistance training program. Before you dive in, you need to do some self-assessing to determine your starting point, and we'll give you the tools you need in the next chapter. But first, let's look at Lynne, our next case study participant, and see how she was able to embrace the StrongPath and reverse the effects that excess weight and sarcopenia were having on her life.

CASE STUDY: LYNNE

At 54, Lynne was sedentary and severely overweight. She is a professional singer, entertainer, and writer. She once lost 100 pounds and then gained them all back. She was mortified by her failure. Her weight became such a burden, she only left home to work. Otherwise, she stayed in and watched television. Lynne said her weight was so bad that she was "hobbling around like a grandma." To compound matters, she also has osteoarthritis and a bad left knee.

Lynne was starting from a much different place than many of the other test subjects. She'd been a member of the spa at the Trump International Hotel and Tower since it opened, but along with knee and back pain, she lacked motivation, so she struggled. She started the test training with a smile, but also with some hesitation. She knew when she came in that the first couple of sessions would be a challenge for her. She had the motivation of her friends and Fred, but she also knew her health and mobility were on the line.

After initial measurements of weight, body fat, strength, flexibility, and cardio, which all showed her to be on the negative side of the scale, Fred and Lynne's trainer knew that any improvement for Lynne would be a great improvement and a movement toward a much healthier lifestyle. Her trainer told her that the first month would be the toughest, as she would be feeling the workouts. He also shared that there would be aches, pains, and tightness, but that she'd sleep better. Lynne knew that while training would be tough, it was going to increase her metabolism and help stabilize her, because she would be using smaller muscles, and as a result of that, she would have less injury and pain.

She and her trainer talked about her diet, and she worked with a nutritional expert. They discussed the importance of the timing of meals, what to eat, what to stay away from, and what to do to counter bouts of inactivity or while performing in shows. Along with the measurements, they also did an assessment of how she was moving, how she was compensating, and an overall attitude, energy, and well-being tally.

When Lynne couldn't get to the gym, or she slipped up on her diet, they had contingencies. She worked out at home and worked on bettering her other meals. She drank a lot of water and kept moving. Her trainer would get feedback from her and keep her entertained as they progressed. In addition, she got homework assignments. She was on it—she never missed a beat. If she came in with a cane on some days, her trainer modified the workout. They also incorporated stretching and core into every workout.

Each week, Lynne's trainer increased resistance as well as reps and sets. They mixed it up a lot, too, with a variety of exercises. Her body reacted well to the challenge. They would do 2 days of strength training a week and 1 day of mobility and pool cardio. In a 5-month period, her movements improved, her aches and pains decreased, and her energy increased, as did her flexibility. Her resistance and weights increased in varying degrees between 50 percent and 75 percent.

As for her strength gains, they started almost every week with her trainer increasing the resistance. He pushed for more repetitions, added another set, and gave her a variety of exercises for the equipment. She got the movements and form down quickly and also knew whenever her trainer increased the resistance or weight. Her trainer checked in to see how she was feeling, while he studied her form and made necessary modifications to ensure a good workout. They've also started adding boxing, swimming, kettlebells, and free-weights, along with functional exercises as her abilities have advanced.

Fear Factor

Lynne joined the test study because she felt challenged. "Fred said to me one day while I was at his house that I was unhealthy and needed to get in shape," she said. "He offered to pay for my strength training, but then added, 'But I don't think you will do it.'" That was the challenge that got her going. Once she went home, however, fear set in. She knew she was in bad shape and that her excess weight and lying around all day were making her depressed. But with the challenge to change came a concern: Failure could follow. And failure was public. "If I didn't keep up," she said, "Fred would know about it." She was terrified that even if she got started, she'd eventually revert to her old ways—she feared humiliation, embarrassment, and physically falling apart.

Biggest Surprise

Lynne took a trip to France while she was well into her training. It was summer and 98 degrees outside. She had to perform on stage, and before strength training, she had been growing exhausted by the performances and regularly struggled to catch her breath. While on location, the heat and normal physical toll was increased, because she had to make her way across an enormous field at a castle—on foot. Looking back at France, had she not been training for 3 months, she wouldn't have been able to walk across the field or pull off the performance. But now she was in great shape! She had shed 25 pounds and tackled what would have once been insurmountable with great ease and confidence. That's what the strength training had done for her. And that trip alone gave her the boost to know she'll keep at it. "It's a lifestyle change for the betterment of my remaining existence, and it must never stop. I've got a lot of work to do and I've made the commitment to do it for the rest of my life," she said. And this surprise attitude adjustment came just a few months into her effort.

The other surprise: She realized no one in the gym was watching or cared!

Benefits

When asked about benefits in addition to strength, Lynne said, "Don't even get me started." She performs better, she's singing better, she was inspired to do a new recording, and she started writing more. Additionally, she feels confident enough to share her journey with her fans and friends. At first, she felt like she didn't want to tell anyone what she was up to in the training department in case she let herself down. But once she saw her success and knew she could keep it going, she began to write and post about the path she'd taken. People wrote back, inspired. Stairs no longer daunted her and her newfound confidence was noticeably apparent!

"It's a lifestyle change for the betterment of my remaining existence, and it must never stop. I've got a lot of work to do and I've made the commitment to do it for the rest of my life."

Your first step: Just walk into the gym. Make that an easy and achievable goal. And go for it.

Words of Wisdom

Lynne has very pointed advice for anyone considering a training program: Do it. She said not to be afraid that someone's going to make you go from zero to one hundred in your first session. She took it very slowly—in baby steps. She went from breathing heavily from just walking down the hall to embracing her trainer and the gym. Your first step: Just walk into the gym. Make that an easy and achievable goal. And go for it.

Mind Games: Steven's Solution

Lynne's story will resonate with many of you out there who fear failure and who struggle with their weight. Fear of failure is much more than fearing that time and money will be wasted. There is that for sure. But the part of fear of failure that makes you queasy is related to being exposed for weakness, uncomfortable awkwardness, appearing unknowledgeable, asking stupid questions, and fearing the loss of respect and esteem of others during the process of failing. The older we are, the more frightening just about any new prospect becomes. We concentrate increasingly on what we do well and avoid what we do not. As the years go by, we stick with the things we've gotten good at over the years. Physical activity is one of those things we avoid. In fact, it is the great tragedy of our time that engaging in physical challenges that could greatly improve our health has become an arena of wholesale avoidance. So, the challenge of shifting gears and getting started is at first psychological. That's what Lynne probably faced long before Fred intervened.

One thing that Lynne had going for her before she got started with her resistance training is that she left the house to work. The call of the stage still moved her. Yes, it provided her with an income, but she also had people showing up to hear her sing. Many of us are moved to work and do things for others we might not do for ourselves. There is a motivation in being called to do something, as it is a great blessing. Fred saw that Lynne's current health and future health were in jeopardy. He called to her. Lynne, in return, is calling to others. She's built a following to help her through her quest for health and so that she can provide motivation

Continued

to those just starting out. She knows what they face and she cares. She calls. She shared and a community began to grow. One important fact to keep in mind on your quest is that motivation need not be wholly individual. Having resolve, doing your best, showing up—all those things are individual. But having the wind at your back because others care—that is what really helps.

The pathway through the inner resistance that Lynne faced is accessed by patient, incremental effort. You will need some simple physical assessments, but many of them can be done on your own. They will get you focused on the first few things that you need to work on. Then, step-by-step, you will quickly begin to build real strength and you will move from success to success. Soon, you will be showing others how to do what you have done and the psychological hurdle will have been left far behind. You need to just get started and break through your resistance and fear. Think about Lynne if you're struggling to do so.

The difference between the power, beauty, and overwhelmingly earthy richness of real-life physical experience as it contrasts to theoretical knowledge or the vicarious "action" of lying in bed watching TV is beyond words.

AN EMAIL EXCHANGE BETWEEN FRED AND LYNNE

Lynne: It's interesting. I am starting to plan my life around my workouts. I found myself saying (at a recent birthday gathering), "I really can't have another drink, I have to work out tomorrow and if I'm slightly out of it, my workout will be inefficient, because I'll be sluggish." My friends exchanged glances. Then laughed until they saw I was serious. Do you realize it's been 16 months since I started this journey? The journey has changed. I am also becoming focused on nutrition. I need to get this weight off, because it's an obstacle in the gym. It's holding me back. How's that for an attitude adjustment?

Fred: Perfect. Our StrongPath view is that it is more important to "get strong" than to be badgered about losing weight. What happens as we get strong is we learn we WANT to lose weight without being badgered by others. It is just what happens.

Lynne: So true! I see it every day: the weakness and subsequent sedentary behavior which, of course, leads to weight gain. I know of few people who sit around all day and don't eat all the time. You do more when you feel physically stronger because you can! There's a certain kind of confidence when you know that you can do more physically. When you work out consistently you understand that pain or muscle exhaustion is something you work through. I might wake up with knee pain, but I know that once I get up and warm up my muscles by moving, the pain dissipates. You only learn that by moving every day, pushing yourself, 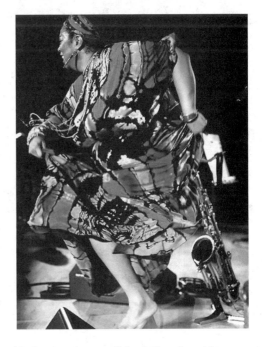 *and never giving up. The old girl would give in, give up. "I hurt therefore I lay around until I'm feeling better." Working out makes me feel better.*

Fred: You have realized one of life's great truths!

Lynne is back and better than ever!

CHAPTER 11

Ongoing Objective Assessments

WHEN TAKING THE StrongPath, it's important to remember that medicine and fitness merge into a whole-life health program and that your individual program needs to be continually assessed. Understanding your physical limitations and strengths, as well as your medical history, will help you identify where to begin your journey. One thing to remember: Don't be in a hurry to get started. Know what you're getting into and know yourself. You are opening an entirely new path in your life; you are not jumping into another here-today-and-gone-tomorrow fad diet or exercise program. Getting on and staying on the StrongPath depends on doing things correctly, not doing things quickly. It also depends on your ability to build a lifelong heath and training discipline that will keep you connected with the best that science and medicine have to offer over time; the StrongPath allows your knowledge of self to expand and strengthen along with your body.

We're going to ask you to put on your management cap as you embark on this journey, so be patient and walk through the steps that will help you get started in a healthy, injury-free way. You will not only be learning how you should begin and what you should do but also how to advise your parents, other family members and friends, kids, and coworkers. Knowledge is power. You want to own and control your journey and your strength training—so learn what you are doing and why you are doing it.

> **Knowledge is power. You want to own and control your journey and your strength training—so learn what you are doing and why you are doing it.**

This chapter will equip you with the tools to help you assess yourself and get assessed by a professional. You will learn about the tools that you need to make wise decisions as you embark on the StrongPath. Most important, you will learn there is no one-size-fits-all approach to health care, diet, or exercise. That is why simplistic enthusiasms and diet approaches not only fail, they can do more harm than good. Instead, we encourage a customized approach and objective tests to help you along the way.

START BY SEEKING MEDICAL APPROVAL

We recommend that you get a physical exam before beginning our plan. Your doctor needs to be a part of your lifelong StrongPath team. If you have chronic conditions or past injuries that need special consideration, you will need his or her input, so you can work within safe parameters. Your physician will also be interested in what you are doing and how your work is objectively improving your overall health.

Your annual physical exam will be an integral part of your ongoing training. StrongPath training is powerful, and it will affect your overall health in measurable ways, so it is also great to know the results of your blood tests and your blood pressure, for example, at the starting point. Most health insurance covers an annual physical exam. If you have not had one in the past year, you should consider making an appointment to do so. Then, by this time next year, both you and your doctor will be able to see what progress you have made. Members of our test groups have been able to drop or decrease blood pressure and other medications as their test results have improved with strength training. Imagine feeling excited to go to your physical exam, because you are looking forward to seeing new test results. This will happen for you, too.

THE ASSESSMENT PROCESS[1]

The assessment process is where you begin to build your plan. It's also the method by which you'll measure progress over time. Measuring your progress will ensure that you're maximizing the results of your efforts and will demonstrate that you are on the right path. There are many specialists you can partner with to help you, including—

- Rehabilitation physicians

- Physical therapists

- Physical therapy assistants

- Personal trainers[2]

THE PHYSICAL ACTIVITY READINESS QUESTIONS (PAR-Q)

You may feel that you are in good health and confident that you are ready to hit the gym. Still, it is worthwhile to pause briefly and use a highly recommended simple tool that has been created to act as a checklist, like a pilot uses before takeoff, to make sure you have not overlooked some important indicators.

The PAR-Q is a short, simple questionnaire that will take you only a few minutes to use. It was developed by the Canadian Society for Exercise Physiology to help you determine whether you might be overlooking any well-known reasons that you should consult with your doctor about before embarking on, or ramping up, an exercise program.

You will find an updated electronic version by visiting this website: eparmedx.com. It will give you your results instantly after you have answered a few quick questions.

You can also find an explanatory video and a link to eparmedx.com on our Strongpath.com website.

FUNCTIONAL MOVEMENT ASSESSMENTS

Everyone needs to be assessed. If 17-year-old superstar college athletes are assessed and revealed to have weaknesses that if not addressed will get worse, you also need to know your strengths and your weaknesses. You should do this early in your process, so that you can push and engage in progressive training. You need to know your limits and the aspects of your body that you need to improve on to find balance. You might have a lower back issue or a knee issue, for example. As such, your workout will need to be intelligently composed with your personal and individual issues in mind. Here's why.

At first glance, the young man in Figure 11.1 looks as fit as can be. He even has a six-pack. But athletes in sports like tennis tend to develop asymmetrically as a result of the demands of the sport. A qualified strength coach would immediately notice the man's powerful left arm and thin right arm. This asymmetry would be addressed with a balanced strength-training program, making his right side's strength on par with his left side. Doing so would benefit his performance on the court, help him avoid injuries, and improve his long-term health outlook.

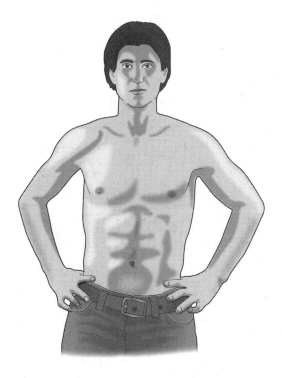

Figure 11.1. Tennis player with asymmetrical arm development.

The bottom line is we are all different and require functional movement assessments. In addition to your physical exam, if you know of a professional at your gym or physical therapist's office who conducts them, make an appointment and have one done. And remember, as you start on the StrongPath, you'll want to do annual assessments with this individual and build on your workout—increasing weight and difficulty as you work to get stronger.

The Science of Assessing

Our friend, strength coach Mike Basgier, assesses top talent entering college sports. They are young and to the average eye appear to be in excellent shape, but coach Basgier sees and measures their failures of symmetry and form that will make each prone to injury if not addressed. He tests and finds strength and flexibility imbalances that need to be addressed in each person's individual workout program. This is all done as a mandatory first step to strength training. These research-based assessment systems are designed to quickly and efficiently note your functional movement issues and to showcase what exercises you will need in your repertoire to address them.

YOUR ASSESSMENT

There are a few types of assessments you might come across as you research getting someone to test you. We've listed a few of the more popular tests:

- For individuals of limited ability because of age, weight, sedentary lifestyle, or other disability, the Short Physical Performance Battery (SPPB) may be the right starting place.

- For most others, the Functional Movement Screen (FMS) is a great assessment tool.

- Some professional team and college sports strength coaches use the more detailed Physical Competency Assessment (PCA) for advanced athletes. If you're at this level, you're beyond what we're talking about in the following pages and probably have your own team of professionals already helping you.

SPPB

The SPPB[3] holds a special place given it has been the focus of numerous studies throughout the international research community. There is a growing body of data that demonstrates the efficacy of the SPPB as an assessment of your current functional movement ability and your future risk of disability onset. Even more important, individuals who work to increase their strength and improve their assessment scores over time enjoy a commensurate decrease in risk going forward. The SPPB focuses exclusively on lower extremity function (leg strength and balance). Research and medical communities have recognized that lower extremity function is an important factor of overall health.

But you may be wondering why physical performance would be predictive of future health risks in older adults. This question was answered specifically in relation to the SPPB in a study published in the Journal of the American Geriatrics Society.[4] The study reveals that your body is the physical evidence of your overall condition at any moment. Physical function measures appear to integrate the effects of aging, disease, nutrition, fitness, and emotional state, yielding a bottom-line indication of your state of health.[5] Dr. Fielding and Dr. Boppart both feel strongly that this assessment should be a natural component of an annual physical exam for everyone age 65 and older. They also believe it should be part of Medicare's annual wellness visit. This would proactively catch and make it possible to address indications of developing functional problems while they may still be simply and inexpensively addressed. Doing so would preserve quality of life and reduce health-care needs and costs. On Dr. Fielding's urging, Steven and Fred will be lobbying Congress to include this assessment as part of the annual Medicare wellness visit.

The SPPB takes very little time to complete and is simple to administer. The National Institutes of Health (NIH) offer online a complete training

CD,[6] including video to demonstrate how to administer the assessments. The assessments can also be downloaded from their website.[7]

The SPPB relates directly to your ability to safely do the activities of daily living. For example, the chair stand test consists of doing squats. If you don't think a squat is something you need to be able to do, remember that getting up off a toilet seat is essentially a squat exercise.

> Greater strength means enjoying independence during more of your life.

Not being able to stand back up after using a toilet is one reason people must enter elder-care centers. Having the strength to get up off the seat is essential for independent daily living. A simple squat and other lower-body exercises build the muscle you need to live independently with dignity. If you learn to safely do your squats with good form, you will get stronger, your next assessment will improve, and you may be able to avoid having to enter assisted living. It is as simple as that. Greater strength means enjoying independence during more of your life.

If getting up out of your easy chair or recliner is challenging, or if when you are walking down the street or at a mall you notice that other pedestrians seem to forever be rushing by, the SPPB is likely the right beginning assessment for you. In addition to what you can find on the NIH website, you can watch the videos we've created on our website, Strongpath.com, to help demonstrate each element of the SPPB assessment, which consists of three kinds of assessments: one for balance, one for gait speed, and a third for your ability to get out of a chair.

FMS

In addition to the SPPB, our StrongPath group went through FMS assessments in Vail before starting our StrongPath workouts. While there, we met some members of the Vail police force and rescue squad. They were strong and young, but they were getting their annual FMS done, too. According to their test results, each was receiving his or her individual exercise counseling and prescription for the coming year, so they would all know how best to refine their workouts to improve and avoid future injury.

The FMS is a well-developed and tested system used around the world at gyms and by strength coaches. It evaluates people on an individual level, allowing them to then develop a strength-training program. Even pro athletes get these evaluations. And they're done quarterly to test, retest, and enhance performance.

What's most important to know about this FMS system is that it's not testing whether you can squat or do a leg raise, it's measuring the quality of each movement—analyzing weaknesses and strengths in *your* body and muscles. We suggest that if you're going to make an expenditure, you go to a good gym with qualified and certified staff and make an investment in an FMS assessment and have one or two training sessions from the personal trainer to get you started. We don't assume you can afford a trainer three times a week. If you can, great, but at a minimum we're hoping you see the investment of the needed $100–$200 to do this as an investment in your future and that you can spend it, get tested, and learn from it before you get started on the StrongPath. A good trainer will be able to look at the strength-training program we provide in the next chapter and see that you get engaged in it in accordance with your functional movement abilities and proper form.

These tests will reveal weakness in, say, one arm as opposed to the other, or whether your back swayed or stayed straight for a push-up.

They will also determine the level of your core strength. This individual opening data will be your reference against which you can test again later to see improvements in your functional movement capacity as well as your strength over time. You can visit our website for resources, where we also include the link to the FMS website[8] that certifies testers and can point you in the direction of someone certified and qualified to help keep you healthy and injury-free in your area.

HOPEFULLY, YOU NOW understand how important it is to assess your ability before you get started on the StrongPath. These tests will not only ensure that you work out safely, slowly increasing the difficulty of your workout, but also will enable you to track your progress over time. Be sure to keep your doctor in the loop. In the next chapter, we'll begin your StrongPath plan and teach you how to get started in the gym. But first, let's meet Gayle, our next case study participant, who was a little resistant initially but soon discovered the benefits the StrongPath afforded her.

CASE STUDY: GAYLE

At 64, Gayle has always thought of herself as a strong and capable person with about 10–15 pounds to lose. As a registered nurse, she works extremely hard in a taxing and physically demanding job. She has never been to a gym, but she spends days on her feet.

Gayle reported initially not losing weight in the program in spite of seeing strength improvements. This is likely due to the fact that those improvements were coming through increased muscle activation and improved technical form with movements that she was not previously comfortable with. Her continued improvement through the middle and later stages of the program were in part due to both of those positive adaptations as well as to likely increases in the size of muscle fibers as she was continually challenged to lift heavier weights.

Gayle saw more modest percentage improvement to her lower-body strength, due to the fact that she already worked at a physically demanding job. She wears a wrist monitor of her steps, and she walks 6–10 miles up and down long hospital hallways every shift. Her improvements in technique will undoubtedly protect her during work hours from potential lifting injuries that might occur as she works with patients.

Fear Factor

The gym wasn't a place Gayle feared. It was, however, a place she didn't like. Though she's committed to it now and enjoys the results of going, she said she still doesn't really like it much. She overcame her dislike by realizing the gym was where success occurred. She briefly tried to work out at home but then realized that the appointment at the gym was critical, because it forced her to stick to her training. What

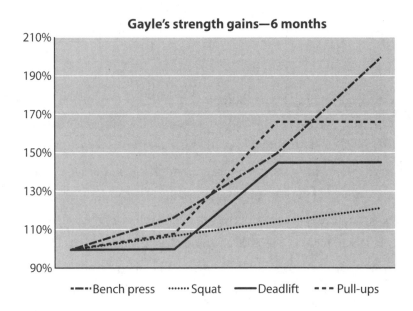

Gayle's strength gains—6 months

- – – Bench press   ········ Squat   ——— Deadlift   – – – Pull-ups

moved Gayle to go to a place she didn't love was working in a job where she was constantly exposed to illness and weakness, because it made her recognize that she needed to avoid that fate. She started to realize that people were succumbing to disease at ever younger ages and recovering from illness at slower rates than seemed logical. That thought motivated her. Instead of just preaching as a health-care provider, she changed her own health by proactively jumping in and doing something about it.

Biggest Surprise

Gayle wasn't surprised that she could dive in and train and accomplish something. She was floored, however, by how fast she saw results. She said she couldn't believe how quickly she increased her strength and saw dramatic improvement in her initial measurements.

Benefits

Already a positive thinker, Gayle found that after training, her posture and overall sensation of movement and walking were completely
different and more powerful. She was impressed by how quickly that
change revealed itself. She said aside from feeling stronger, she felt
pride in her accomplishment and impressed she'd changed her body.
She found she slept better because she'd worked out so hard. And
although she didn't feel any reduction of stress in her 13-hour shift job,
she did sense improvement in managing the stress, mostly because "I
felt a greater sense of confidence in my physical ability and felt inner
strength I didn't have before."

Words of Wisdom

Structure and a dedicated schedule are what kept Gayle going. Knowing that there were days in the week when she could escape and do
her workout motivated her. She said she also felt
tracking her improvement was a motivating factor
for someone like her, who wasn't a "gym person"
to begin with. Her advice: Trust it and try it. The
rewards will appear almost immediately. "You can
do your job better and feel better and healthier, plus
know you're protecting your future."

> Trust it and try it.
> The rewards will
> appear almost
> immediately.

"I work in a busy telemetry ward for seriously
ill patients aged 20 to over 90. The ones under 40 who come in are not
generally fit or muscular. They are not strong. They are in the hospital
often because of gastrointestinal issues, for example, and many are also
addicted to painkillers. The few who are fit are suffering from some odd
medical issue like blood clots in their legs and lungs. These patients
get treated and released pretty quickly. The older ones, as they age,

> "It is always an inspiration when I get an older person who has some strength and sparkle left. Their chances are always much better for an improvement in health than that of the patient in the next room who is unwilling to try to move. Be one that sparkles. The difference is priceless."

are weakened by the addition of weight, which complicates their medical problems. The ability for them to achieve a healthy outcome becomes more remote. Some are what we call 'frequent flyers,' because they have medical conditions that will not get better without serious behavior modification, which they do not undertake. As a result, they return episodically. It is always an inspiration when I get an older person who has some strength and sparkle left. Their chances are always much better for an improvement in health than that of the patient in the next room who is unwilling to try to move. Be one that sparkles. The difference is priceless."

Mind Games: Steven's Solution

There's a great lesson in Gayle's experience (who is, by the way, my wife). When tackling just about anything, we often show up to a new situation with a preexisting attitude. Gayle did. She didn't like the gym. Even after the training period ended, she thought she could get it done at home. The good news, as she learned, and you will too, is that attitude is not fixed. Do not believe that any negative attitude you might have in the beginning is destined to remain an ongoing barrier to your success. Attitudes shift with new experiences, with social influences, and with your own motivation. Knowing this will help you accomplish something.

Your attitude is simply part of where you begin. Where you go from there can change, and you can overcome that initial notion. An attitude will seem like a huge factor if you give it a lot of attention and struggle to hold on to it. Alternatively, your attitude will wink out of existence during the time you focus on engaging in movements with full attention. It will change. That's because attitudes are emotion-fueled thoughts rather than fixed realities. New experience, new shared perspectives with others, and successful new achievements will give birth to new and different attitudes.

Part of this shift comes from habit. As we have said, strength training needs to become a habit for you. Structure and routine build habits, and habits are the key to long-term success. When older portions of our brain take over and launch behaviors, such as getting to the gym at set times 3 days a week or doing squats before breakfast without the draining need for a conscious decision to do so on each occasion, then we add a powerful ally that replaces that most unreliable character: willpower.

As you progress, all the little wins will start to emerge. You may notice these successes as you get stronger by an increase in the amount of weight you can lift or the number of stairs you can climb, but these improving statistics are not why you are working. The real payoff is when suddenly you notice that your posture has changed, that you feel strong, and that your walk expresses a certain greater confidence that communicates your new strength. This will cause others to look at you in a different way. This is a powerfully moving and meaningful success, the kind that bit by bit influences your attitude. Things that loomed large at first as obstacles get cast in a new light by such experiences.

One-Year Update

Beginning with 50 pounds of weight, after 12 months of training, Gayle can now deadlift 165 pounds. This has made it much easier for her to move heavy patients in hospital beds. Her opening bench press has improved from 30 pounds to 70 pounds, greatly improving her upper-body strength. And she now smiles and looks forward to going to the gym.

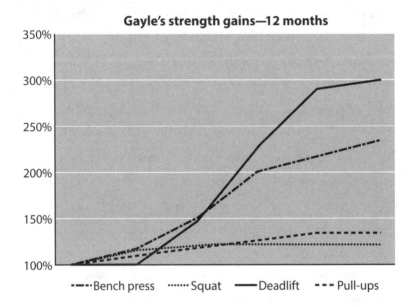

CHAPTER 12

Working Out: Building Your StrongPath Plan

ONLY 21.9 PERCENT of all adult men and 17.5 percent of all adult women in America participate in strength-training programs. Those that need strength training most do it least. In addition, the "prevalence of strength training among men and women decreased significantly as age increased."[1] The figures for those doing more than minimal strength training are a fraction of those cited here. Those doing the minimum recommended sessions twice a week get weaker more slowly than those doing no strength training. Thus, virtually everyone embarking on the StrongPath is a beginner and not truly acquainted with the kind of strength training that can increase strength as you age. If you are 40 or older, chances are you used to be stronger and fitter than you are today. That has been the trend. But from your first workout going forward, that fate-filled trend is going to change.

> 66
>
> Virtually everyone embarking on the StrongPath is a beginner.

OUR APPROACH: IT IS ALL ABOUT STRENGTH

There is not just one way of gaining strength, but there are essential fundamentals. In this chapter, we will explain the fundamentals and how to get started. Each one of you is starting from a unique point and set of personal circumstances. So you will be learning to engage in exercising all your muscles in a way that continually assesses your abilities and works at the level that is right for you, every time you exercise. This process is simple, and you will use it to automatically adjust your workout as you grow stronger. Don't be in a hurry or jump ahead in the process. Strength is success, and it will come most quickly with focused, steady effort.

A Few Key Terms

- *Rep* is short for "repetition." When you do a push-up, you lower yourself and push yourself back up to the position you started from. You just did 1 rep. Do it ten times, and you have done 10 reps.

- A *set* is a group of reps. Your workout plan will call for you to do 15 reps, for example, of a light weight to begin with. This will be your 1st set. Increase the weight and do 10 more reps. This will be your 2nd set.

- Between sets you will *rest* and give your muscles a chance to recover before doing another set. Rest periods should be from 1 to 2 minutes between sets, with a high number of reps using a lighter weight. Rest time will increase to 2 to 3 minutes between sets when fewer reps are done with heavier weight.

BEGIN IN A GYM

StrongPath training is designed to rapidly increase your strength by initially stimulating more efficient motor unit recruitment, teaching your existing muscle cells to engage and work. This begins to happen from your very first workout, and you will reach a peak of percentage strength gains during the first 2–4 months.

Strength gains from increased muscle mass will begin to occur simultaneously, but more gradually. This means that if you spend money on home equipment for strength training, like dumbbells or resistance bands, you will be growing out of them quickly and having to buy more constantly. At a gym, you will just use the next heavier weights or adjust the resistance setting on the machine you are using.

If you have minimal equipment, the only way to increase the work is to do more repetitions. Over time, every exercise will become a form of endurance rather than strength training and that is not our goal. At a gym, you will also find the equipment you need for a rotating full-body workout at different resistance levels. You will see the importance of this as we get into the details.

Plus, you will learn a lot just being in a gym. You will find trainers that you can hire to teach you proper form, and many gyms offer classes that teach you to use the equipment properly.

> **Strength training is such powerful medicine that it represents a rapidly growing frontier for health care.**

In addition, the social aspect of a gym is very positive, and you are safer with others nearby rather than being alone. If you have a Medicare Advantage Plan, there is a good chance that you are one of the fourteen million that qualify for a free pass to over thirteen thousand gyms nationwide. Check silversneakers.com to learn more.[2]

And for those of you not on Medicare, the YMCA is a great low-cost organization that traditionally has promoted resistance training.

Strength training is such powerful medicine that it represents a rapidly growing frontier for health care. You will want to be connected with a facility that places you with people and equipment that will evolve with new discoveries. Our website will also keep you abreast of what to look for and try based on scientific research and new discoveries.

YOUR SCALE WILL NOT REVEAL HOW MUCH YOUR BODY IS CHANGING IN THE BEGINNING

It is common for weight to show little change during the first few months of strength training. This is because your body composition is changing. You may lose 4 pounds of fat and gain about the same amount of weight in lean mass. So stepping on the scale will not reveal that much has happened, but you may find that you had to tighten your belt by a notch. Your thighs may have become a little tighter and harder, as they slide into your jeans more easily. And your arms are firming, and even your face is beginning to change as your strength grows.

A WORKOUT DIARY IS A MUST

Your workout diary is where you will keep the personal workout log sheets we provide. You can find these log sheets in the Resource section of Strongpath.com. With our guidance, you will learn to work out all your muscles in a rotation that keeps your body growing progressively stronger over time. The template we provide will make it simple to jot down the exercises you will be doing and to record the weight and how many repetitions you complete. There is also a cardio exercise section designed to record distance and time.

Copies of the template can be printed out as you need them, and we recommend that you keep the hard copy in a file or binder. There

STRONGPATH

Workout Log   Date _____

Plan	65%	15		75%	10		80%	8		85%	5-6		90%	3-4	
Strength Exercise	Int.	Reps	Wt	Int.	Reps	Wt	Int.	Reps	Wt	Int.	Reps	Wt	Int.	Reps	Wt	**PR**

Int. – intensity   Reps – repetitions   Wt. - weight

Cardio exercise	Time	Intensity	HR	Time	Int.	HR	Time	Int.	HR	Time	Int.	HR	Time	Int.	HR

HR – heart rate

are many electronic apps, but our experience is that over time problems with changing technology, software, and formats end up causing the loss of your history and progress. Your diary will be the historical record, the book, of your experience. You will want to keep both statistics and your personal notes about breakthrough moments and how your self-image and confidence evolve as you progress. Use the blank back of the page to jot down important experiences and realizations. They will have an enduring value.

Your collected series of executed workout plans will become the chronological book of your achievements as each workout session adds a new page. A sample log appears above, to give you an idea of the records you will be keeping.

THE SURPRISING ROLE OF "PERSONAL RECORDS"

People who are used to gyms and exercise frequently are heard saying, "I made a PR today in bench press." A PR is a personal record, and it means that person lifted more weight in a particular exercise than ever before in his or her life. PRs have a surprisingly important role in your exercise program. The personal record is uniquely important to your health and happiness, because keeping such records provides a powerful motivation to work harder, challenge your body more, and become stronger. You will smile every time you enter a new PR.

It is important to emphasize here that lifting the same weights for the same number of repetitions, over and over, might maintain your strength. But this will not increase your strength, and you will not achieve the maximum benefits from your exercise. Individuals at a gym that are stuck in a repetitive cardio exercise routine with perhaps some light resistance work will tell you how long they have been coming to the gym. They will not have a mental sense of progress in terms of PRs that hallmark increasing strength and ability.

Keeping a log of personal records inherently keeps us focused on steady improvement. It is a normal, natural incentive to do better and to try new ways to challenge different muscles to increase stability, power, and range of motion. Having a written PR history means you no longer will be depending on a vague and changing sense of how you feel as the indicator of your fitness progress. The record of your progress will be right there before you in solid, immutable facts. As a result, you will *know* you are on the right track. All ambiguity is removed. Knowing you are on the right track in life is the best guarantee that you will stay on the right track.

Each new PR is solid proof of progress. Giving every PR an honored and special place in your workout history and your life will be a continuing powerful incentive toward becoming the absolute best you can possibly be. This is why we encourage you to keep these records. We want you to have a constant motivator toward success.

In the next chapter, we will dive into our full-body training approach. But first, let's look at our next case study, where we will meet Wendy, who had a lifelong struggle with her weight before embarking on the StrongPath.

CASE STUDY: WENDY

At 44, Wendy was overweight. She always knew she had to lose weight. She spent a lifetime dieting—hopping from one fad-dieting plan to the next. Since she was an athlete in high school and college, and didn't shy away from yard work over the years, she assumed that despite the ups and down on the scale, she was strong. It wasn't until her first session with our trainer that she realized she wasn't.

Wendy was an interesting case study. She had no formal training upon entering the study, which meant that she had a pretty intense learning curve in terms of getting down all of the lifting techniques. Additionally, Wendy is an example of a study participant whose work and travel schedule interfered greatly in her regular attendance to training sessions. There were some weeks when she could make her three training sessions and others when she had to do the best she could to come in at all. Some of her results indicate a period of prolonged absence, with an upturn more recently as she could accommodate more training sessions into her schedule.

Wendy clearly showed her greatest gains in the lone strength exercise that did not involve moving her own body weight. Shortly before the writing of this report, she stated she wanted to lose some excess body weight. Accomplishing this would more than likely also significantly contribute to improvements in her ability to move additional weight.

While certainly not her favorite lifting days, Wendy did show impressive improvements to her lower-body strength and stability. The strength she gained there will be immensely beneficial in her next stage of training when she works on losing excess body fat. Her improved stability and increased strength allowed her to move heavier weights and contributed to her improved ability to reach her fitness and wellness goals as evidenced in Figure 12.2.

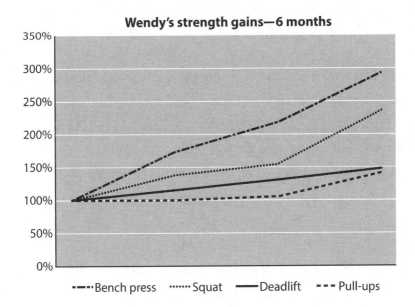

Fear Factor

While Wendy was excited to have this opportunity to train for our experiment, it wasn't until she got in the car to go to her first session that panic set in. "I was so nervous," she said, "I almost cancelled." She knew an assessment of her fitness level awaited her upon arrival. In her head, that meant a hard-core stress test and lots of people at the gym staring at her. She said she almost turned the car around. Wendy said there were a few thoughts that kept ringing through her head:

- She had tried everything before. Why would this work when nothing else had?

- She was embarrassed by the thought of standing in front of other people.

- She'd gained weight over the years and was worried the stress test would be unbearable.

All her fears dissipated once she got through her initial meeting with Cullen. The stress test and assessment were, in her words, simple. While she knew she had a long way to go, she realized immediately that it was neither embarrassing nor scary. Once she went to train, she quickly knew it was something she would be able to do.

Biggest Surprise

Wendy learned immediately just how weak she actually was. Her grip strength, balance, and flexibility were tested during the assessment. She went to do a lunge with one knee touching the floor. She got down into the position just fine, but then she was floored by what happened next: She couldn't get back up. She was mortified by how weak she was. She had to use a bench and a free hand to lift herself up. That was her aha moment. "I didn't know whether to laugh or cry," she said. "I could have run out the door. Instead, I said to myself, 'I don't want to live like this.' I knew at that moment I needed to change so that in 20 years when I dropped my keys, I could pick them up again." Wendy viewed her weakness that day as pure motivation.

Benefits

While there's no finish line to this process, and the most obvious benefit to strength training is strength and a change in body shape, Wendy's extra benefits were substantial. She feels healthier, and life is easier.

Carrying a suitcase through an airport or doing yard work is easy now, and the change is noticeable. She doesn't sweat a flight of stairs anymore either. The successes are so small, yet so enormous. Since embarking on the StrongPath, she hasn't gotten sick once.

Words of Wisdom

Wendy wants anyone considering a strength program to know that getting started, at any level, is no big deal. She also wants people to understand that overall happiness and strength go hand in hand. Her lifelong half joke of thinking she'd be fat and happy was misguided. Strong and happy was the combination she was now embracing. Weight and strength are unrelated. She is no longer using weight as an excuse to not train. Wendy states that once you get started, "it's very easy to succeed. Just show up. It will all get better."

> "It's very easy to succeed. Just show up. It will all get better."

Wendy discovered another wonderful surprise available to those who have little or no experience with strength training. She discovered how quickly the human body can make life-changing strength gains. Within a few months, strength can literally be doubled and all manner of activity that seemed lost and gone forever is easily within reach and even fun again. This is just the beginning of a completely different and better life that lies ahead in terms of health span and quality of life for Wendy. She has noticed how confidence surges along with strength gains. Initial fears and worries fall away quickly. Your sense of self is powerfully influenced by bodily changes and physical success. This allows your mind to see the path and understand how to continue to advance. The experience of progress is always a surprise. From the cellular level up, much more is happening than can ever be understood. We become more alive and an inexpressible joy rises.

Mind Games: Steven's Solution

Wendy's fear of going to the gym the first time is more than common. Fred says he is still surprised how many of his closest friends and colleagues admit feeling they cannot do what he does, because they are afraid of going to a gym. The reasons vary from fear of being seen in workout clothes to being afraid of having other people watching them to a fear of just appearing weak. In each instance, you can hear that initial tinge of panic Wendy felt and expressed.

Take heart in Wendy's experience. Her anticipation of getting started was nearly debilitating. The reality of getting started was no big deal, and the real lifelong rewards open to her now are incalculable. Her experience of beginning with a competent objective strength and mobility assessment gave her the confidence she needed to begin the strength training.

We are all built differently. More important, few of us truly know how fit we are. We are all a collection of memories about ourselves that are likely out-of-date. We remember what we could once do, which is often quite different from what we can safely do now. If we are not regularly involved in some activity that tests the range of our abilities, then we really don't know our own physical capacities. Simple assessments reveal this and open our eyes. Current data gets us started at the right level, taking old injuries or specific weaknesses into consideration. Get started. Your fears will evaporate and be replaced with a wonderful new you.

One-Year Update

Wendy had an intensive 6-month period of demanding travel with her work during the year and was not able to meet her training schedule on many occasions during that period. Still, beginning with a dead lift capacity of 125 pounds, after 12 months of training, Wendy can now deadlift 205 pounds. And her beginning bench-press capacity of 40 pounds is now 125 pounds. The only setback she experienced was that her beginning pull-up strength of 95 pounds dropped to 85 pounds. But she plans to remedy that by resuming her regular sessions.

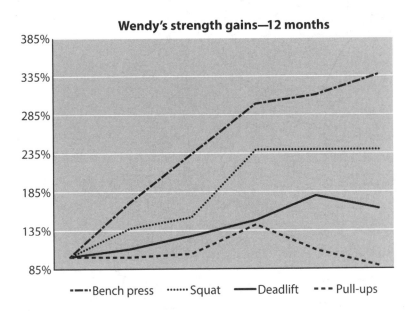

Wendy's strength gains—12 months

CHAPTER 13

Your Full-Body Training Approach

In this chapter, you will learn how to incorporate the StrongPath into a balanced, full-body approach that you can customize to meet your goals and needs. We will take you through your warm-up and show you how to gauge the intensity of each session. Then you will learn the weight-resistance exercises, followed by the full-body circuit, where you will work each muscle group for maximum benefit. We will also show you how to rotate your sessions every 2 weeks, so that you can set yourself up for success on the StrongPath.

CARDIO: YOUR WARM-UP

A 5- to 10-minute warm-up on common gym equipment like a treadmill, elliptical machine, or rowing machine is a great way to get your whole body warmed up for the resistance training you will be doing. The older you are, the more important it is to factor this into your routine. Start slowly, particularly if you are a beginner, and then pick up the pace. How will you know what pace is right for you? Your heart rate will be a primary personal reference and guide. Being aware of

> Being aware of your heart rate as you exercise is a simple but powerful form of real-time biofeedback.

your heart rate as you exercise is a simple but powerful form of real-time biofeedback. It is a tool that makes it possible to calibrate every cardio exercise experience to your fitness level.

LET INTENSITY BE YOUR GUIDE

Intensity is a key reference. To increase your strength and health effectively, you must learn to measure the intensity of your workouts. There are two ways you can do this.

The first way works great for cardio exercises. It is by monitoring your heart rate. Cardio exercise machines at gyms typically display your heart rate as you exercise. You can also buy a basic heart-rate monitor wristband for around $40. Check Strongpath.com for current recommended options. Figure 13.1 shows the recommended intensity levels by age, so that you can aim for your target zone each time. The second way works for resistance training by determining what percentage of your maximum effort you are exercising and will be explained in the next section.

Gauging Intensity Using Your Heart Rate

Your heart rate is expressed in beats per minute. Your heart-rate intensity is a percentage of your maximum recommended heart rate. To stay in the recommended zone, you will be working out at less than 100 percent of the maximum rate at which your heart can beat safely.

As you can see in Figure 13.1, the recommended maximum heart-rate levels in terms of beats per minute decrease with age, and the Mayo Clinic provides guidance for the level of intensity you should work out at according to your fitness level. If you are wanting to achieve moderate exercise intensity, you should strive to be in the 50–70 percent range during your workouts. For a more vigorous exercise intensity, you should be in the 70–85 percent range.

Maximum and Training Recommended Heart Rates by Age

Maximum Heart Rate		Intensity % - Beats Per Minute				
Age	Beats Per Minute	50% Rate BPM	60% Rate BPM	70% Rate BPM	80% Rate BPM	85% Rate BPM
20	200	100	120	140	160	170
25	195	98	117	137	156	166
30	190	95	114	133	152	162
35	185	93	111	130	148	158
40	180	90	108	126	144	153
45	175	88	105	123	140	149
50	170	85	102	109	136	145
55	165	83	99	116	132	140
60	160	80	96	112	128	136
65	155	78	93	109	124	132
70	150	75	90	105	120	128
75	145	73	87	102	116	124
80	140	70	84	98	112	119
85	135	68	81	95	108	115
90	130	65	78	91	104	111

Figure 13.1. Maximum Training Recommended Heart Rates by Age

The Mayo Clinic advises, "If you're not fit or you're just beginning an exercise program, aim for the lower end of your target zone (50%). Then, gradually build up the intensity. If you're healthy and want a more vigorous intensity, opt for the higher end of the zone."[1]

You can apply this to a 10-minute cardio warm-up on a treadmill, for example.

Look at the age column on the chart and find the number closest to your age. Let's say you are 50 and have not been exercising, but you are not ill or suffering disability. Then a moderate warm-up will be appropriate. Read the 50-year-old line to the right and find the beats per minute recommended for 50 percent intensity and you will see that it is 85 beats per minute. That is your target range for a moderate warm-up. Then look for the 60 percent and 70 percent numbers and note them all on the cardio section of your workout log. If you will be doing vigorous warm-ups, note the corresponding heart rates for 70 percent, 80 percent, and 85 percent in the cardio section of your workout log. These target numbers will not change for some time, so once noted you will not have to do this again for a while.

Light to Moderate Warm-Up

At the gym, if you are that 50-year-old who has not been exercising, 50 percent intensity or 85 beats per minute is your first target. Start slowly on a treadmill and walk while holding the metal sensors that will report your heart rate. Over a minute or two, find the pace that keeps your heart rate at or around 85 beats. If at any time, even if after exercising for only a minute or two, you find you are laboring hard and your heart rate is increasing above this level, even at a very slow pace, it is time to stop. Note how long you were able to walk and record it in your workout log. Rest and repeat the effort if you can. You may need to build up your stamina slowly in the beginning. Next time you may be able to do a little more, and so the process begins. We all must start where we are at and work from that point. If you have walked at 50 percent intensity for 5 minutes and feel fine, increase your pace to 60 percent intensity for 3 additional minutes. Then, if you are feeling up to it, you can increase your pace to 70 percent intensity for the final 2 minutes if all is going well.

Vigorous 10-Minute Warm-Up

If you have been exercising and are fitter, you are probably acquainted with treadmills and ready for a more vigorous warm-up. You can begin walking and gradually increase your pace until you are working at 70 percent of your maximum heart rate. Then maintain it for 5 minutes. You can increase your pace until your heart rate reaches 85 percent of your max heart rate and continue at that level for 1 minute. After a minute, reduce your speed until your heart rate drops back to 70 percent of your max for 1 minute. Then increase it back up to 85 percent for a minute. And then take it back down to 70 percent for the remaining amount of time. Adding a couple of minutes of higher-intensity effort pulls your fast-twitch muscle cells into play. This is an important element of strength training, and it does not significantly occur if you exercise below 75 percent of your max heart rate, regardless of how long you exercise.

After you are warmed up, you are ready to go. As you get fitter, you will naturally be increasing your speed and/or incline on a treadmill to reach the same heart-rate levels as your body strengthens and becomes more efficient. Be sure to note these changes as they occur in your workout diary.

Also, try not to get into the habit of always warming up on the same machine at the gym. Mix it up. Use the same heart-rate formula on an elliptical machine, rowing machine, stair climber, or other cardio machines. Each uses a variety of different muscles in different ways, and the variety will work in your favor. When you are warming up, work on maintaining good posture (head up, shoulders back), so that your core muscles engage and benefit from your warm-up exercises too.

Gauging Intensity in Weight and Resistance Exercises

Your 1-repetition max is the most weight you can lift one time. When you work to lift the most you can one time, you should be working at 100 percent of your maximum intensity. Your 10-rep max is the most weight you can lift ten times in a row. When you work to lift the most you can ten times in a row, you should be working at around 75 percent of your maximum intensity. When you are doing 15 reps, you should be working at around 65 percent of your maximum intensity.

Look at Figure 13.2 and find the number of repetitions you will be doing. Note the corresponding weight/intensity level, and you will begin to see how the chart works. Strength coaches have devised simple charts like this that are indicative of what your ability at different levels of intensity will likely be.

Such charts are a guide developed primarily as a result of professional observation rather than scientific testing, so there is some variation in charts from different sources, but the resulting numbers over time are similar. They work pretty well for beginners as well as for those with strength-training experience. The numbers in Figure 13.2 are used by Mike Basgier, the head basketball strength and conditioning coach at James Madison University. We have added comments and explanations to help you navigate the chart.

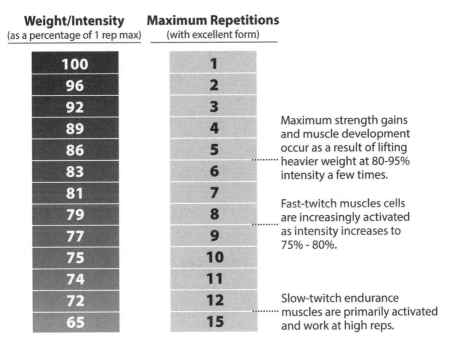

Weight/Intensity (as a percentage of 1 rep max)	Maximum Repetitions (with excellent form)	
100	1	
96	2	
92	3	
89	4	Maximum strength gains and muscle development occur as a result of lifting heavier weight at 80-95% intensity a few times.
86	5	
83	6	
81	7	
79	8	Fast-twitch muscles cells are increasingly activated as intensity increases to 75% - 80%.
77	9	
75	10	
74	11	
72	12	Slow-twitch endurance muscles are primarily activated and work at high reps.
65	15	

Figure 13.2. The Role of Resistance Exercise Intensity on Muscle Fiber Adaptations[2]

In the same way we used different heart rates to compose a cardio warm-up exercise with variable intensity, we can now use the chart to approximate the intensity levels to a weight-lifting exercise. We will be able to program each specific exercise to build endurance, strength, muscle, and bone mass by working at different intensity levels. You will know the intensity level by knowing the number of times you can lift, pull, or push a given weight. The amount that you can do will change progressively and increase in terms of either the reps you can do or the amount of weight you can manage. Each can be matched to the chart, so you can determine the relative intensity level you are working at. Doing this makes it possible to calibrate your every resistance-exercise experience to your fitness level.

> **Your body needs time to adapt to new challenges.**

Never start by trying to find the most you can lift at one time. It is not safe to jump right into the highest-intensity challenge. Your body needs time to adapt to new challenges. On each occasion that you work out, start with the low weight and high rep sets. This provides a muscle-specific warm-up that makes working with heavier weights in later sets safer.

THE FIRST TIME YOU ADD AN EXERCISE TO YOUR WORKOUT

The Dumbbell Bench Press

A little trial-and-error testing will let your body determine the right weights to use. Select a set of dumbbells you think you can bench-press 15 times or more. Err on the side of too light. Lie on your back on a flat bench and press both weights straight up at the same time. Try and do 15 reps.

If you could not do 15 repetitions at the current weight, go down to the next smaller weights. Conversely, if you could have done more repetitions, go up to the next heavier weights for the next set. Rest a minute or two and retest another time, and you will find the right weight for you to begin working out at 15 reps.

If the weight that was right for you was 15 pounds in each hand, for example, then bench-pressing 15-pound dumbbells 15 times for you on this occasion will be exercising at around 65 percent intensity. Sixty-five percent is a good intensity level to activate your endurance muscles and to work on perfecting your form and the rhythm of your breath.

Doing 15 reps using 15-pound dumbbells is 1 set. Enter this data into your workout diary, as shown in Figure 13.3.

Strength Exercise	Sets	Reps	Wt	Sets	Reps	Wt	Sets	Reps	Wt	Sets	Reps	Wt	Sets	Reps	Wt	PR
Dbell press	1	15	15													

For beginners, plan to work up to doing 3 sets of each exercise and increase the weight for each set as you are able the first couple of months. For example—

- Do 1 set at 65 percent intensity, which is the weight you can work with for 15 reps.

- Do 1 set at 75 percent intensity, which is the weight you can work with for 10 reps.

- Do 1 set at 80 percent intensity, which is the weight you can work with for 7–8 reps.

Record the actual number of reps you manage in your diary as illustrated in Figure 13.4.

Strength Exercise	Sets	Reps	Wt	Sets	Reps	Wt	Sets	Reps	Wt	Sets	Reps	Wt	Sets	Reps	Wt	PR
Dbell press	1	15	15	1	10	17.5	1	8	20							

Those of you who have already been exercising regularly can add a 4th set at 85 percent intensity, which is the weight you can work with for 5–6 reps. Those of you who are more advanced and have been doing significant weight training can add a 5th set at 90 percent intensity, which is the weight you can work with for 3–4 reps.

Each of you will have tested at different levels and the level that you begin with will quickly evolve as you grow stronger. Now you can compose a workout plan for this exercise that will keep you on track to grow stronger over time. When you do a specific exercise again, check what you could do the time before. For example, if with the same weight you did 15 reps before, see if you can now do 16 or 17 reps. If so, note it in your workout log. Then next time this exercise comes around, see if you can do 15 reps of the next larger weights.

This makes it possible for everyone to continually customize their workout in a way that one-size-fits-all workout plans never can. It will make all the difference in the results you achieve, because it will keep pace with your growing strength and ability and lead you to each next step up as soon as you are ready.

KEEP YOUR FOCUS ON YOUR GROWING STRENGTH AND CONTINUALLY NUDGE IT FORWARD

This is an important part of your lifelong health care. Learning to read and challenge your body by working at the intensity levels that will continually improve your health and fitness puts you in a position to take responsibility for maintaining your training. If you dive in, the necessary learning will come quickly as you develop your diary and get acquainted with a collection of basic exercises that you can expand on over time.

Written instruction and still images do not adequately communicate exercise movements that may be new to you, so plan to review the movements of exercises on our website and make it your constant companion in this process.

SCHEDULE

You will need to get to the gym 3 days a week for 45–60 minutes. It is best to schedule a non-exercise day between your workout days if possible. It is also helpful if you can dedicate a recurring time on your calendar for your workouts that are consistent, like Monday, Wednesday, and Friday at 7:00 a.m. The more you make your workout time a priority, the better. You want to build a solid habit, so if it's Monday, Wednesday, and Friday from 7:00 a.m. to 8:00 a.m., you have committed yourself. All you have to do is show up and do your best to avoid any scheduling conflicts.

BEGINNING THE FULL-BODY CIRCUIT

There is a universe of possible exercises, so it is important to remember what your primary objective is. We want you to develop the whole-body strength that translates into a superior ability to easily maintain your mobility, perform the tasks of daily living, and stay engaged in the wonderful world of physical activities that you love throughout your life. Life is full of demands for compound movements where your legs, arms, core, hands, and feet all work simultaneously. Therefore, the strength you seek is not the narrow ability to flex isolated muscles to the exclusion of others; rather, it is to develop a system-wide musculature that is practiced at working together as a competent symmetrical whole. So it is important to build your exercise program on the four pillars of essential compound movements (hip hinge, squat, bench press, and the pull) that are invariably part of life's physical challenges.

Today, we are more sedentary than ever before. We sit through most of the day. We recline in the evening, watching TV. As we gain weight, we spend more time in bed, watching TV. Work commonly occurs in an office, sitting slumped in a chair at a desk. Very simply, this leads to chronic back pain. All the time sitting with poor posture or in bed wastes the muscles responsible for keeping our spines steady and aligned. Our fast-twitch muscle cells, which are critical for actions as simple as climbing stairs or standing up from a chair, waste away first.

These muscles need an exercise movement and a resistance challenge that will get them engaged and doing their job competently again.

The first movement you must master is the hip hinge, which Tony Bonvechio refers to as "exercise's most important motion."[3] We have chosen two variations of hip-hinge exercises for different levels of beginning ability: kettlebell swings and barbell dead lifts. Kettlebell swings are for the moderately fit who need to master the movement, and the barbell dead lift is for the more advanced who have mastered the hip-hinge movement and are ready to begin heavier progressive training. The equipment commonly found in gyms has a different weight range to allow for progressive training as you strengthen. Kettlebell sets usually begin with just a few pounds and graduate up, so that most individuals will be able to find a comfortable weight to practice and become acquainted with the hip-hinge movement.

For those who find bending and lifting challenging with body weight alone, we recommend beginning to strengthen key muscles on the seated leg press machine before moving on to kettlebell swings. The leg press machine will allow you to strengthen your legs, beginning at much less than body weight, and you will be able to increase resistance progressively until you are ready for a more complete body movement. If bending over to lift triggers back pain, you will need supervised rehabilitation and instruction to get started safely.

Video demonstrations of each of these exercises are found at Strongpath.com along with a presentation of the basic hip-hinge movement and some warm-up exercises to start with to get used proper back posture and hip motion.

We will use the basic progression of intensity as before to create our workout plan for any one of the three exercises. As you begin, plan to work up to doing 3 sets of an exercise and increase the weight for each set as you are able the first couple of months. For example—

- You can do 1 set at 65 percent intensity, which is the weight you can work with for 15 reps.

- Then do 1 set at 75 percent intensity, which is the weight you can work with for 10 reps.

- And then do 1 set at 80 percent intensity, which is the weight you can work with for 7–8 reps.

Record the actual number of reps you complete in your diary, as shown in the sample chart in Figure 13.5. As you gain strength and find that you can do more reps with a given weight, progress to the next largest weight and record the number of reps you can do with it. Work with it until you can do more than the target number of reps at each intensity level and then work your way up in weight once again.

Strength Exercise	Sets	Reps	Wt	Sets	Reps	Wt	Sets	Reps	Wt	Sets	Reps	Wt	Sets	Reps	Wt	PR
Kbell swing	1	15	5	1	10	8	1	8	10							

For those who have already been exercising regularly, add a 4th set at 85 percent intensity, which is the weight you can work with for 5–6 reps. For the more advanced who have been doing significant weight training, add a 5th set at 90 percent intensity, which is the weight you can work with for 3–4 reps.

The next movement to master is the squat. The squat is critical to balance and leg strength. It also is important for your fast-twitch muscle cells. Doing squats properly will make you strong and steady on your feet, which is important at any age. Squats will strengthen your lower body, your core, and upper body as you add weight. Squats will also make you feel lighter on your feet. You will be able to rise, move, and turn with confidence, and you will be better able to catch yourself if you stumble, avoiding a fall.

A proper body-weight squat without additional weight can be

challenging for those who have not been exercising. Depending on your fitness level, you may need to begin with a quarter or half squat for a few reps until you begin to strengthen. Then progress to a full-range-of-motion body-weight squat.

For those of you who are more advanced, once you master the movement at full body weight, you can advance to doing goblet squats with a kettlebell or a dumbbell held close to your chest. Once you have worked through the progression of weights available, you will be ready for barbell squats.

We will use the basic progression of intensity as before to create our workout plan. For beginners, plan to work up to doing 3 sets of an exercise and increase the weight for each set as you are able the first couple of months. For example—

- Do 1 set at 65 percent intensity, which is the weight you can work with for 15 reps.

- Do 1 set at 75 percent intensity, which is the weight you can work with for 10 reps.

- Do 1 set at 80 percent intensity, which is the weight you can work with for 7–8 reps.

Record the actual number of reps you manage in your diary, as shown in the sample chart in Figure 13.6. As you gain strength and find that you can do more reps with a given weight, progress to the next largest weight and record the number of reps you can do with it. Work with it until you can do more than the target number of reps at each intensity level and then work your way up in weight once again.

Strength Exercise	Sets	Reps	Wt	Sets	Reps	Wt	Sets	Reps	Wt	Sets	Reps	Wt	Sets	Reps	Wt	PR
Goblet squats	1	15	10	1	10	12.5	1	8	15							

For those of you who have already been exercising regularly, add a 4th set at 85 percent intensity, which is the weight you can work with for 5–6 reps. For those of you who are more advanced and have been doing significant weight training, add a 5th set at 90 percent intensity, which is the weight you can work with for 3–4 reps.

If you are advanced enough that you are already doing barbell back squats, check the form points in our videos for this exercise and then apply the progressive intensity approach described in the preceding pages to your program to ensure that you are being incrementally challenged and have not settled into a fixed routine.

The third of our four essential compound movements to master is the bench press. This may seem at first to be an exercise that strengthens your arms primarily. But, when the bench press is properly done, with feet planted firmly flat on the floor, straight down from the knee or a little behind the knee, shoulder-width apart, it becomes a full-body compound movement. It strengthens muscles from your grip, wrists, forearms, triceps, shoulders, chest, and back, right down through your legs to your feet.

Once again, it is essential to master the movement before you handle much weight. In this exercise, it is best for everyone to start by doing the dumbbell press, because it is important to work on left-right muscle and strength symmetry from the beginning. Most everyone is left- or right-handed, and it is important to begin working with equal weights in either hand to build balanced strength and stability. Choose the weight that your weaker arm can do for 15 reps to begin with and work up from there over time at the pace that your less proficient limb can manage. In 4–6 months, you will be surprised to find that both have become much stronger and much more similar in ability.

In most gyms, dumbbells are in graduated sets, starting at just a few pounds and going up to very heavy weights, so everyone can find a good starting place. In the weight room, the rack will usually start at 5 pounds. If you need a light weight to start, you may find some starting as low as 2 pounds in an area of the gym that has exercise classes that use lighter weights.

For beginners, plan to work up to doing 3 sets of each exercise and increase the weight for each set as you are able the first couple of months. For example—

- Do 1 set at 65 percent intensity, which is the weight you can work with for 15 reps.

- Do 1 set at 75 percent intensity, which is the weight you can work with for 10 reps.

- Do 1 set at 80 percent intensity, which is the weight you can work with for 7–8 reps.

Record the actual number of reps you manage in your diary, as shown in Figure 13.7.

Strength Exercise	Sets	Reps	Wt	Sets	Reps	Wt	Sets	Reps	Wt	Sets	Reps	Wt	Sets	Reps	Wt	PR
Dbell press	1	15	15	1	10	17.5	1	8	20							

For those of you who have already been exercising regularly, add a 4th set at 85 percent intensity, which is the weight you can work with for 5–6 reps. For the more advanced who have been doing significant weight training, add a 5th set at 90 percent intensity, which is the weight you can work with for 3–4 reps.

The fourth movement to master is the pull. This fundamental movement balances the growing strength and muscles you will be developing by doing press exercises like the bench press.

Pulling is another movement that you need for many of the activities in your daily life. Pulling also demands system-wide, coordinated strength. Think of opening a heavy doorway to enter an office building on a windy day. This action requires a solid stance and a sturdy core, along with the needed arm, shoulder, chest, and back strength to pull with. There are also occasions when you need to pull yourself up. Having the pull strength to do so is an important part of maintaining confidence and independence long term. In reflecting on what strength you need to develop in each of the four fundamental movements you will be working with, do so in the context of your body weight. Your ability to move your own weight is essential for quality of life and securing your long-term independence. This is a big job, yet it is the job your body was designed for, and it has an amazing ability to adapt and rebuild itself accordingly when adequately challenged to do so.

There are two machines at the gym that allow us to progressively develop our pulling strength, beginning with light loads and high reps as we have done in the other basic movements. These are the seated cable row machine and the seated lat pull-down machine.

Once again, plan to work up to doing 3 sets of an exercise and increase the weight for each set as you are able the first couple of months. For example—

- Do 1 set at 65 percent intensity, which is the weight you can work with for 15 reps.

- Do 1 set at 75 percent intensity, which is the weight you can work with for 10 reps.

- Do 1 set at 80 percent intensity, which is the weight you can work with for 7–8 reps.

Record the actual number of reps you manage in your diary. As you gain strength and find that you can do more reps with a given weight, progress to the next heaviest weight and record the number of reps you can do with it. Work with it until you can do more than the target number of reps at each intensity level and then work your way up in weight once again and record your findings, as shown in Figure 13.8.

Strength Exercise	Sets	Reps	Wt	Sets	Reps	Wt	Sets	Reps	Wt	Sets	Reps	Wt	Sets	Reps	Wt	PR
Seated Row	1	15	20	1	10	25	1	8	30							

For those of you who have already been exercising regularly, add a 4th set at 85 percent intensity, which is the weight you can work with for 5–6 reps. For those of you who are more advanced and have been doing significant weight training, add a 5th set at 90 percent intensity, which is the weight you can work with for 3–4 reps.

SPEND YOUR FIRST WEEK OR TWO AT THE GYM GETTING ACQUAINTED

If you are new to the gym, don't try to learn all the exercise machines, the proper use of weights, and test your strength as instructed the first time you go to the gym. Instead, start by getting acquainted with the treadmill, learn how to get it to report your heart rate and how to change your pace to move your heart rate up and down to the target rates. Once you are proficient at that, begin to test your strength as instructed and record the results on a workout log sheet.

Over the course of several days, learn the different movements we have covered for the full circuit training and test what weight you can manage for each of the different exercises. When you have collected these notes on worksheets, you will be able to build your opening workout plan.

STRONGPATH

Workout Log

Date _____

Plan	65%	15	75%	10	80%	8	85%	5-6	90%	3-4

Strength Exercise	Int.	Reps	Wt	Int.	Reps	Wt	Int.	Reps	Wt	Int.	Reps	Wt	Int.	Reps	Wt	PR
Kettlebell swing	65%	15		75%	10		80%	8								
actual																
Lat pull down	65%	15		75%	10		80%	8								
actual																
Seated cable row	65%	15		75%	10		80%	8								
actual																

Cardio exercise	Time	Int.	HR	Time	Int.	HR	Time	Int.	HR	Time	Int.	HR	Time	Int.	HR
Treadmill	5 min.	50%		3 min.	60%		2 min.	70%							

On the workout log sheet, available for free download on our website, use the white columns to write your planned workout. In the light grey column, record your actual results. These may differ, because you may find that you can do more than your plan calls for in terms of reps at a given weight. This means that next time at the gym, as that exercise comes around again in the cycle, you will want to try the next heavier weight and see how many reps you can do with it. In any exercise, when you do more than you have ever done before, check the PR box and circle your new personal record.

CREATING A ROTATING 2-WEEK FULL-BODY WORKOUT PLAN

Blank versions of the workout logs in this section can be downloaded from our website. They will be integral in helping you structure your rotating workouts. The exercise log that follows is a sample of one day's workout for a moderately fit beginner. It contains exercises for two of the four primary movements. You will use a sheet like this every other day that you work out. You will use the second workout sheet after it with exercises for the other two primary movements that you will implement every other day.

STRONGPATH

Workout Log   Date _____

| Plan | 65% | 15 | | 75% | 10 | | 80% | 8 | | 85% | 5-6 | | 90% | 3-4 | |

Strength Exercise	Int.	Reps	Wt	Int.	Reps	Wt	Int.	Reps	Wt	Int.	Reps	Wt	Int.	Reps	Wt	PR
Kettlebell swing	65%	15		75%	10		80%	8								
actual																
Lat pull down	65%	15		75%	10		80%	8								
actual																
Seated cable row	65%	15		75%	10		80%	8								
actual																

Cardio exercise	Time	Int.	HR	Time	Int.	HR	Time	Int.	HR	Time	Int.	HR	Time	Int.	HR
Treadmill	5 min.	50%		3 min.	60%		2 min.	70%							

Figure 13.10. Workout Log, Day 1

Print another log to record your activity on day 2, as shown in Figure 13.11.

STRONGPATH

Workout Log   Date _____

Plan	65%	15		75%	10		80%	8		85%	5-6		90%	3-4	

Strength Exercise	Int.	Reps	Wt	Int.	Reps	Wt	Int.	Reps	Wt	Int.	Reps	Wt	Int.	Reps	Wt	PR
Leg press machine	65%	15		75%	10		80%	8								
actual																
Dumbbell bench press	65%	15		75%	10		80%	8								
actual																
Dumbbell shoulder press	65%	15		75%	10		80%	8								
actual																

Cardio exercise	Time	Int.	HR	Time	Int.	HR	Time	Int.	HR	Time	Int.	HR	Time	Int.	HR
Treadmill	5 min.	50%		3 min.	60%		2 min.	70%							

Figure 13.11. Workout Log, Day 2

You will alternate between these sheets every time you go to the gym, so you can work the full circuit. Go back to Figure 13.1 on page 191 to look up the recommended heart rate for your age at the different intensity levels listed. Record this on the Treadmill row, which is your first warm-up exercise. Take this log with you to have as an easy reference guide at the gym.

Once you have tested the weight you can manage for 15, 10, and 8 reps, fill in the boxes in the weight box that you plan to do. Every time you work out, if you can do a few more reps than the plan, note that you did so in the actual row. Remember that you will find similar prepared sheets on our website for different starting levels that take into account the need to use less advanced or more advanced equipment.

Remember: Form is critical. When you learn proper form, your body will become toned as you gain strength and prevent injury. Proper form is the "chisel" with which you will sculpt your new physical form.

> **"**
>
> **When you learn proper form, your body will become toned as you gain strength and prevent injury.**

There are, of course, tens of thousands of possible exercises, but we live in a truly wonderful information age. To get acquainted with proper form for virtually any exercise, simply search the Internet; for example, search for "proper form kettlebell swing video," and you will find a variety of good trainers demonstrating and explaining good form for that exercise. You can access the videos at the gym on your smartphone or electronic pad. If you do a Google image search, you will find examples of proper form you can print out if you prefer.

The following list of points will help reinforce the important points about proper form:

- No one spontaneously begins to exercise with proper form; there is a lot to learn.

- Incorrect training technique can lead to sprains, strains, and fractures.

- There is no safe way to engage in serious strength training that does not include learning right form from the very beginning.

- You will grow into the shape and form in which you exercise.

PROPER BREATHING TECHNIQUE

Now that you've learned proper form, you should focus your attention on proper breathing. Proper breathing is critical to your health and safety during weight lifting. Your breath oxygenates your system and removes waste products. But that is just the beginning of its importance. Conscious control of your breath and the focus of attention powerfully influences your autonomic system.

> **Proper breathing is critical to your health and safety during weight lifting.**

To follow the proper breathing technique—

- Inhale when you lower a weight and exhale as you lift. Different exercises require different patterns of movements, so remember that the general rule is to exhale with exertion when you either push or pull against resistance.

  It is a common error for strength-training beginners to hold their breath when lifting. This causes dangerous spikes in blood pressure. It also causes abdominal pressure that can lead to hernias.

- Focus your attention on the sound of your breath and the bodily sensation of each exercise movement.

Do not think while you are lifting. Let go of any anxious thoughts or worries. Don't let your attention dart off to the mirror to see if you look good or to notice who is paying attention to you or to watch TV. No multitasking is allowed during your workout. The capacity of your nervous system to communicate is not infinite. That's why we don't text and drive. Movement is a demanding, complex skill. Try watching an action movie and typing at the same time. Or walk up to a free throw lane and start worrying about where you left your cell phone while trying to shoot hoops.

Dividing your attention destroys your ability to move fluidly and purposefully. So, give yourself a break from distractions. You are trying to learn something very important and very difficult to do precisely right, and this requires focused attention. Notice how often your mind is not where your body is. You are not present with your body in space or time if you get lost in a past regret, worry about the future, or are texting or talking on the phone. Your attention easily drifts away and is somewhere else entirely. During your workouts, stay focused. Moving and lifting with good posture and form are not something that you can learn if your attention is elsewhere.

Listening to the sound of your breath puts your attention in the present moment, where the action of lifting is occurring. In this mode, your unconscious command of the extraordinarily complex task of movement is learned and refined automatically. When mindful, you will improve most quickly; your body will respond and grow anew in millions of ways at the cellular level. Only in this mode will you do your best and develop most quickly.

And trust us on one more point. Every human being looks their best when they are focused in the present on doing something well. Proper breathing and present-minded focus of attention will increasingly add the benefits of mindfulness to your life with every workout.

For a complete supporting multimedia reading and visual presentation of this chapter's components, visit our website at Strongpath.com. On our website, you will find a world of ongoing strength-training possibilities, such as demonstrations on how to use the charts and workout log sheets and exercise video demonstrations, which can be accessed on a smartphone or tablet

> Proper breathing and present-minded focus of attention will increasingly add the benefits of mindfulness to your life with every workout.

and taken to the gym. You will also see and hear from others on the StrongPath who will show you what they are doing and how they fit their training into their busy lives.

In the next chapter, we will learn how to feed our muscles with a balanced diet. However, before we move on, let's look at our next case study, where we will meet Fred's sister Stephanie, who chose to embrace the StrongPath and a healthier diet.

CASE STUDY: STEPHANIE

When Stephanie Shay turned 55, she had a big birthday party to celebrate. Later, when she looked at the photos from the evening, she was devastated. "I thought I was beautiful," she said. "Then I looked at pictures and realized I looked just awful."

Stephanie stepped on the scale and realized that, without noticing, she'd crept up to 207 pounds. A few things had contributed to her weight gain over the years. In 1980, she gave birth to her first daughter, Melissa, who was born with Down's syndrome. Care was difficult and the situation was upsetting for Stephanie, who says she became depressed as she struggled to raise her baby. Stephanie's second daughter, Sarah, was born 3 years later. In the ensuing years, when Stephanie's mother was diagnosed with cancer, Stephanie quit working in real estate to care for her ailing mom. Unfortunately, she had spent so much time caring for others she hadn't taken much time to care for herself.

Stephanie had been a size 8 for much of her younger years. She never worked out a day in her life, ate a lot of fast food, and didn't pay much attention to her weight. She knew her knees and hips ached, but didn't think that it had to do with the weight inching up on her. Her health was solid and she never had any problems.

The year she turned 55, she went to see Fred. Inspired by Fred's workout, and at his urging, she decided to start doing strength training and to lose 50 pounds. Fred encouraged her to keep her weight loss steady and to not lose more than 1 pound a week. He said once she got the excess weight off, she'd be amazed by how great she felt. He told her to think of her journey as a lifestyle change rather than a diet.

Stephanie got a trainer and started going to the gym five times a week doing cardio to warm up and then began her strength training. Three years later, Stephanie is 40 pounds lighter, a size 10, and a regular at the gym.

Stephanie is grateful to Fred for pulling her aside that day and encouraging her to work out. She also wishes her mother had been able to take care of herself the same way that Stephanie had finally learned to do. "I think she would have lived longer," she said.

Vegetables were suddenly a part of Stephanie's diet in a way they had never been before. She stopped eating the fast food and pasta, which she used to love, and other than some chicken, she stopped eating meat. She said it doesn't make her feel great and she wants to put things in her body that nourish her.

"Once in a while, I see a slice of cake and think, 'I want to have that,'" she admits. And she does. "But then, I get right back on it. I'd like to lose some more weight, but most importantly, I've learned to maintain."

But something else profound and important happened in addition to her body changing. Stephanie's confidence level soared. She went back to school and regained the real estate license she let lapse so long ago. She'd thought about it over the years but wasn't sure anyone would want to buy a house from her. She didn't think she had the ability to sell anymore.

"It was a self-esteem thing," she said. "Once I felt physically stronger, I decided: I can do this now." And did she.

She has sold about one house a month since getting her license and has new clients coming in often. She attributes the success to the boost she gets from working out. "I have a ton of energy. I have my coffee in the morning and I'm off and running all day."

CHAPTER 14

The Final Critical Habit: Feed Your Muscles

ALL THE FOCUS today on weight loss has led us to equate *dieting* with *health.* The notion that you can starve your way to health has led many to adopt dangerously misguided diets. Starving through dramatic calorie reduction is not the way to deal with sarcopenia. Sure, if you are overeating like most people today, then managing caloric intake is smart. But simplistically restricting calories is not the answer. Being too restrictive and eliminating the key nutrients needed to support lean mass is not the answer and often makes things worse. Weight loss is harmful when the weight you are losing includes the muscle and bone you need to be healthy and strong.[1]

To be healthy, you must habitually participate in adequate aerobic and strength training. In this context, "good nutrition" is a diet that adequately supports healthy vigorous activity and the process of body recomposition, reducing body fat and adding muscle. Diet and exercise programs designed to work in tandem are the way toward real long-term health. The key is not dieting but instead feeding,

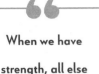

> When we have strength, all else falls into place.

fueling, and building your body in a positive, scientific way to maintain energy and increase muscle mass as you tackle strength training. If you are overweight and pursue strength training and eat scientifically, traditional dieting is not needed. You will slowly and steadily get where your genetics designed your body to be at its healthiest. And there is a key component of good nutrition that plays a central role as you work to build strength and reshape your body in favor of lean mass: protein.

When we have strength, all else falls into place. Strength indicates body composition, the amount of muscle and bone you are made of as compared to fat.[2] Your weight does not.

FIRST: STOP PARTICIPATING IN THE MADNESS

Many of us want to lose weight fast. The quicker and easier the promise of lots of pounds just melting away, the more enticing. But the truth is that losing too much weight too fast is bad for our bodies. The ads that suggest we can and should lose 10 pounds in 10 days are actually hurting us.

Part of the problem is that the Federal Food and Drug Administration (FDA) has no power to regulate fast weight-loss claims. Weight-loss supplements do not need any FDA approval before being advertised. As a practical matter, sellers can make any claim they want.

RAPID WEIGHT-LOSS SCHEMES ADVANCE SARCOPENIA

According to Kathleen M. Zelman, MPH, RD, LD, on WebMD, "Severely slashing calories may lead to weight loss, but the lost weight includes precious muscle and lowers metabolism. Drastic calorie restriction also causes a shift toward a higher percentage of body fat, which increases the risk for metabolic syndrome and type 2 diabetes."[3]

Not only that, if you lose weight quickly, you may gain it back and more. *The New York Times* did a report on rapid weight loss as part of an examination of the show *The Biggest Loser*—in which participants drop hundreds of pounds in a short period of time. At the end of the show, most contestants gain it back because of the damage they've done to their metabolism. The article in *The New York Times* explained that a person's body actually fights to regain that fat.[4]

Rapid weight losers thus become rapid weight gainers, even though they continue eating a low-calorie diet. Rapid weight loss responds to evolution by changing the body, so it can exist on less food. When starved, our bodies throttle back our need for energy.

Rapid weight loss makes us worse off in terms of sarcopenia and, even worse, changes our bodies, perhaps forever, into more efficient fat producers. We know individuals who travel once a year or more to spas that promise the loss of "8 pounds in a week" at a cost of $8,000 or so for the week. Just think: An entire high-profit business exists by charging huge weekly fees to make customers less healthy by destroying the muscle and bone critical to health and happiness and by turning their bodies into fat-creating machines.

There are people who take this journey annually, sometimes more than once a year. Even the few who adapt to continuing and increasing starvation and avoid weight rebound become "skinny fat." That is, they are thinner but their body composition has less mass and a higher percentage of fat after every such session. They are heading down the Frail Trail.

> **"**
>
> None of the rapid weight-loss diets warn us of the life-and-death risks that such diets create.

Remember: None of the rapid weight-loss diets warn us of the life-and-death risks that such diets create, and there is no requirement that those offering such diets have to prove that their plans are safe and effective. Don't trust these diets if you truly want to be healthy.

THE POWER OF PROTEIN

Mobility, function, and metabolism are all affected by age, and protein has a fundamental effect on these aspects of health. Protein and exercise can help slow down aging. Why? What is it about protein that is so critical to our health and strength?

Protein is an incredibly powerful nutrient that can signal the body to build new structures and tissues, including muscle. It has many other benefits, too. Proteins in the body have very important jobs. Among them are sending messages to the body to produce muscle fibers, blood cells, and hormones. It also takes a lot of energy to digest protein, so you can eat more of it without gaining weight. Finally, protein tends to make us feel full, which reduces our appetites.[5]

Douglas Paddon-Jones, PhD, is a leading expert in scientific nutrition. He is a professor in the Department of Nutrition and Metabolism at the University of Texas Medical Branch and has done extensive research into sarcopenia and strategies to combat fat gain and muscle loss—particularly by addressing people at risk of losing muscle and function with aging. Dr. Paddon-Jones's research identifies what is occurring inside the muscle (from a mechanistic and signaling approach) and then investigates muscle mass and strength outcomes. His objective is to slow down muscle loss—with a focus on how nutrition affects the issue. His words and research provide the keystone for building a nutrition plan that will work with your exercise regimen to make your future health the best it can be.

Dr. Paddon-Jones urges people not to wait until later in life to adopt the protein-focused framework he recommends. The message is to get into the habit of "consuming an adequate amount of high-quality protein at each meal, in combination with physical activity."[6] He wants people to begin thinking about muscle health while they are in their 20s—to get ahead of the progression brought on by aging.

How Much Protein Do We Need to Fight Sarcopenia?

There has been a common flaw in recommendations for daily protein intake. The error lies in the fact that eating the right amount of protein is not adequately described in terms of a daily dose. It is important to distribute protein well at each meal. Many Americans eat enough protein daily, but they do so in a way that makes a large portion of the protein they eat unavailable for muscle growth and repair.

According to Dr. Paddon-Jones, "To really turn on the potential for muscle building acutely after a meal, it takes about 20 to 30 grams of protein to do so."[7] So the first question is not whether we eat enough protein in a day. Rather, do we eat protein in portions per meal that activate and support muscle repair and growth? A bowl of oatmeal with milk might have 10 grams of protein in it. But 10 grams of protein, for an older adult, doesn't do much to build and repair muscle. If you're a breakfast skipper or you just have toast or a sweet roll with coffee, you never get the protein in the morning that you need during the time of the day you are probably most active. If you exercise strenuously in the morning, it makes matters worse. If lunch is heavy in carbohydrates and fats and does not have the 20 grams of protein needed to feed your muscles, they continue to starve and waste away as the hours pass. If later in the day you eat more than 30–35 grams of protein in a single meal, your body does not then "catch up" nutritionally and use it all to repair and grow muscle. Your blood will have all the protein it can use at one time toward muscle repair and growth once you have consumed 30–35 grams of protein. The chemical signal will be given that it is "full" of protein, at which point your body will work to burn off the excess and convert the remaining protein into fat and store it. You may have eaten in one meal as much or more than the daily Recommended Dietary Allowance for protein, but your muscles could only take advantage of 30–35 grams, and you have missed your daily nutritional need for protein by a long shot.

Dr. Paddon-Jones stated, "We knew from previous work that consuming 30 grams of protein—or the equivalent of approximately 4 ounces of chicken, fish, dairy, soy, or, in this case, lean beef—increased the rate of muscle protein synthesis by 50% in young and older adults. . . . We asked if 4 ounces of beef gives you a 50% increase, would 12 ounces, containing 90 grams of protein, give you a further increase? In young and old adults, we saw that 12 ounces gave exactly the same increase in muscle protein synthesis as 4 ounces."[8]

Dr. Paddon-Jones recommends habitually building your breakfast, lunch, and dinner around 25–30 grams of high-quality protein and performing physical activity soon after a protein-rich meal.[9]

The more seriously you exercise, the more important it becomes to eat this way. The Recommended Dietary Allowance for protein is 0.8 grams of protein per kilo of body weight per day, but in recent years there has been a move to target intakes between 1 gram and 1.5 grams per kilo of body weight per day, especially as we age.[10]

A study published in the *American Journal of Physiology–Endocrinology and Metabolism* revealed how dramatically different outcomes can be when there is ample protein in the diet. The protein was unevenly distributed throughout a day, but given that there was much more of it, the amount consumed at different meals more often was enough to trigger muscle synthesis.[11]

Changes Began Happening Fast

After just 4 days, researchers found that those members of the study, ages 52–75, who ate double the Recommended Dietary Allowance of protein increased their rate of protein synthesis. This is because they were building more muscle due to a change in diet alone.[12]

This initial response to diet alone is relatively short term, so eating ample protein alone is not an adequate long-term strategy for staving off sarcopenia.[13] Rather, it is an example of how ready your body is to improve and grow healthier given what it needs nutritionally to work with. Combine the stimulation of challenging cardio and resistance exercise with this approach to diet and the signal and response between diet and exercise does continue long term.

What Happens When Protein Is Missing?

Perhaps lunch was a salad with plenty of dressing, a generous serving of french fries, and a soft drink. How does your body respond? A study found that if individuals overate in terms of calories but consumed a low amount of protein (5 percent of calorie intake) "more than 90% of the extra energy was stored as fat." Yet "with the normal and high protein diets [15–25 percent of calories from protein], only about 50% of the excess energy was stored as fat."[14]

"Resting energy expenditure responded differently to low vs. high protein intake. Neither resting energy expenditure, nor lean body mass increased in the low protein group. In contrast, the accretion of lean body mass in the normal and high protein groups was the principal contributor to the increase in resting energy expenditure."[15]

Good nutrition providing ample protein powerfully affects metabolism and body composition. When these dietary principles are combined with a well-designed regimen of cardio and strength training, the results are like nothing you have experienced before.

How Much Protein Is Too Much?

There is always a tendency to think that if something is good for you then more must be better. Don't get bit by this kind of mania (especially when powdered protein supplements are involved, which make it easy to consume abnormal quantities). Concerns about excessive protein are valid. Processing excessive amounts of protein can produce ammonia. Ammonia is toxic, particularly to the central nervous system. We excrete the excess ammonia as urea in our urine but there are limits to our ability to do so. It is possible to consume more protein than our body can deal with.

A study in the *International Journal of Sport Nutrition and Exercise Metabolism* titled "A Review of Issues of Dietary Protein Intake in Humans" addressed the debate concerning the safety and validity of increased protein consumption for weight control and muscle synthesis.[16] They noted that much of the advice to consume diets high in protein has been given by some health professionals, the media, and popular diet books in spite of a lack of scientific data on the safety of increasing protein consumption at the time. Their study found that very high-protein diets "on the order of 200–400 grams per day, which can equate to levels of approximately 5 grams of protein per kilo of body weight may exceed the liver's capacity to convert excess nitrogen to urea."[17] The study recommends that maximum protein consume approximately 2–2.5 grams of protein per kilogram of body weight per day. Of course, if you have a medical condition that has compromised your ability to excrete urea, then you must consult with your doctor for individual advice.

What Is High-Quality Protein?

High-quality protein contains all the essential amino acids your body needs. Our bodies can produce some but not every kind of amino acid. The amino acids we cannot produce are called essential amino acids, and we rely on our diet to provide them.

Animal sources of protein—meat, fish, poultry, eggs, and dairy products—tend to deliver all the amino acids we need.

Some of these high-quality proteins, particularly in processed and prepared foods, are not the best ways to get the protein you need, because they come with high amounts of saturated fat, salt, or sugar. So, it is important to not just look at the protein content but to also keep an eye on what else comes in the "package." For example, eating small amounts of processed meats regularly is linked to increased risk of heart disease. Each product has its own combination of ingredients that make them different from fresh meats, such as sodium and nitrite preservatives, high salt, smoking, and high-heat processing. Just 1.8 ounces of processed meat per day (about one hot dog) increases the risk of heart disease by 42 percent and type 2 diabetes by 19 percent.[18]

Protein sources like grains, fruits, vegetables, nuts, and seeds can provide substantial amounts of protein but tend to lack one or more essential amino acids. Vegetarians need to be aware of this and should make an extra effort to see that they create meals that deliver all of the amino acids they need daily. Keep an eye on leucine content. Animal proteins provide higher levels of this key amino acid, which is not as plentiful in plant-based proteins.[19]

Whey protein isolate or soy protein isolate with all essential amino acids are available at most every grocery store these days. These are a quick and simple way to make a drink with 25–30 grams of protein. But don't get the idea that good nutrition is only about protein and that you can live on protein shakes. Your basic plan for a proper diet should be composed of meals with whole foods. That said, these protein isolate powders offer an interesting opportunity, because they differ from whole-food sources of protein in the time it takes before they make amino acids available in the bloodstream to support muscle synthesis.

TIMING IS IMPORTANT

Protein consumed as meat, eggs, dairy, poultry, or fish appear as amino acids in the blood 2 hours or more after you consume them. You can support a strength-training workout triggering well-timed muscle synthesis by eating a meal that includes 25–30 grams of protein 90 minutes before you work out.[20]

Drinks made from whey or soy protein isolate powders appear as amino acids in the blood within 10–20 minutes after consumption. This makes them very useful if your workout cannot be timed well in relation to a meal. A protein shake with 25–30 grams of protein consumed 0–60 minutes after you work out will put the amino acids in your blood when your body is looking for them and can best use them toward muscle synthesis.[21]

GETTING IN TUNE WITH YOUR BODY

We have learned to respect how different human beings can be in terms of our reaction to different diets and why in the end there is no correct diet for everyone. When Steven emerged from his sudden heart surgery, detailed bloodwork was done. The results were awful. His cardiologist began questioning him in detail about his diet. His wife, Gayle, is a vegetarian. To make things simple when meals were made at home, he had been eating what she prepared for herself. What was finally determined was that the high proportion of carbohydrate calories he was eating were a problem for him. So, he changed and began consuming more poultry and fish primarily and over several months his bloodwork improved significantly. Then it occurred to him that Gayle's bloodwork should be checked too, since they had been eating the same things. She got the full battery of tests, but her results were great. Her diet works just fine for her. This was a real eye opener. She began strength training about 3 years ago and is careful to get the protein she needs each day. Her strength increased rapidly as she participated in the test group, and her bloodwork continues to be excellent.

How does something like this happen? The lab work they had done determined what two APOE genes they each carried. Every person gets one from their father and the other from their mother. Gayle has two APOE3 genes. Steven has one APOE3 gene and one APOE4 gene. Carriers of the APOE4 gene have higher levels of total cholesterol and plaque in their arteries, leading to increased risks of cardiovascular disease, stroke, and dementia and Alzheimer's disease.[22]

So, we each may be made with surprising differences, some of which we may have become aware of and some of which we may not yet be. In addition to physical assessments and medical exams and tests, Fred has developed a simple way to follow and reflect on his diet and how different ways of eating affect him. And Steven finds it an interesting way to bring enough focused attention to the process to yield a lot of personal aha moments. He sees that Fred's technique for engaging in an ongoing personal discovery process is a positive and productive way to take full advantage of his own intelligence and powers of observation, and so can you.

FRED'S MIRROR TECHNIQUE

Many nutritionists advise us to keep a food diary and record everything we eat. The idea is that we will learn from the diary what to eat and what to avoid as well as have a better understanding of just how much we are eating. This is a great idea, except that we slip and often fail to actually do it. There is a much easier way to obtain the same information and effect, which we call the "mirror technique."

To do this, buy yourself a quality digital scale that will report your weight in pounds and tenths of pounds. Then procure some dry erase markers. Weigh yourself every morning at the same time. It's easiest to remember to do this immediately upon awakening. Next, enter each morning's digital weight with a dry erase marker on the mirror in your bathroom. Seeing the previous entries on the mirror will remind you to weigh yourself first thing.

You will soon have a day-by-day record of your weight. Unusual weight increases or decreases will stand out and cause you to think, *What did I do and/or what did I eat yesterday to cause that change?* Then you can write down in small writing by the increased/decreased weight entry what you did the day before that made a difference.

You will become very conscious of your weight and what habits affect your weight with literally no effort. And, more important, you will have a record of what affects your weight instead of someone else's theory of what should affect your weight. After even a short period, such as a month of keeping this record on your mirror, you will have learned a lot about your body and its response to diet and activities.

Of course, after a couple of weeks, you will reach the bottom left side of your mirror and will need to erase these entries and start again at the top. Before erasing these entries, record a few simple things you have learned in small writing at the very top of the mirror, and add a little entry regarding how and why your weight evolved during these weeks. Note the trend. Soon, you will develop an intuitive feel for how your body responds to different foods.

When Fred practiced the mirror method, he learned the following things about himself:

- Stay away from bread, sweet rolls, and dinner rolls. Bread is generally consumed before a meal when you are hungry, so it is easy to eat quite a bit of it. He learned early on to avoid all forms of bread, even in sandwiches, because it always seemed from the outset that bread added 0.5 pounds or more to the morning weigh-in.

- Pasta has an adverse effect on his weight. Pasta for dinner has from the beginning seemed to add close to a pound to the next morning's weigh-in, which is unfortunate, because he loves pasta, but it is what it is.

- Fred also avoids fruit juices, energy drinks, and soft drinks. They are full of sugar, and he gains weight whenever he drinks them.

- He's learned to eat potatoes and white rice sparingly. These carbohydrates add weight to his body.

- For snacks during the day, apples are ideal. Honeycrisp apples are tasty, full of fiber, and seem to have a rapid impact on his appetite. They also appear to have no adverse impact on his weight.

- Almonds are another great afternoon snack that boosts his energy and does not seem to affect his weight.

- He does not eat dessert. In fact, he avoids candy and sugar as much as possible.

- Oddly, with Fred, it does not seem to affect the early morning weigh-in if he has a vodka or two the night before. Wine, however, does seem to adversely affect his weight, so he has learned to limit his consumption of wine to avoid putting on excess weight.

- Six ounces of protein at dinner—chicken, shellfish, or fish— favorably affects the morning weigh-in.

- A well-marbled, properly portioned steak has less impact on his weight than one would think. It has a little more impact than fish and chicken, but not a lot more, even though it has much more fat.

- Green vegetables, such as broccoli and Brussels sprouts, have a favorable impact on his weight.

- Homemade clear broth-based soups are great. They are mainly water and can be made by removing a lot of fat. And they can be made with turkey legs, chicken, and a lot of vegetables that he might not otherwise eat.

Fred is not a nutritionist, although he and Steven have researched nutrition and training extensively for this book. He's just sharing what he has noticed over the years, tracking his weight and comparing it to what he ate or drank the night before.

Try the mirror method and see what you can learn! In addition to supporting an increased knowledge of favorable and unfavorable diet items, the mirror system, over time, gives us insight into other aspects of health and weight control. Seeing your weight recorded every single day creates a broad and useful awareness and understanding of how different types of exercise and intensity of exercise affect your weight. For example, you will develop an understanding of how different types and intensity levels of cardio training translate into increments of body weight. The effect of missing a day or two is driven home to you, tending to reinforce exercise as a habit.

Finally, having displayed before you every day a graphic history of your weight over periods of time is of great importance. You learn early that "starving" yourself by skipping meals is a terrible way to try to control weight. You will see that a quick 5-pound weight loss from severe calorie deprivation makes you feel good early on, but always results in an equally rapid gain of the lost 5 pounds. As we have noted earlier, rapid weight loss signals to our old genome that "winter is coming and food will be harder to come by," which will drive our bodies to conserve fat and energy.

On the other hand, we learn from the daily mirror record that slow weight loss results in plateauing, with the body losing 2–3 pounds and then "adjusting" to the new weight over a week or so. It becomes very easy to stay within a pound of a new target weight. It is empowering to understand your body. This knowledge will enable you to control your weight by developing a personal sense for what is going on.

THE TRUTH ABOUT SUPPLEMENTS

None of the billions of dollars in supplements sold in the United States can fill the role of strength and aerobic training of adequate intensity that is required to defeat sarcopenia. A Harvard Medical School

Special Health Report titled "The Truth about Vitamins and Minerals"[23] informs us that—

- About half of Americans routinely take dietary supplements, the most common being multivitamin and multimineral supplements.
- There is no compelling evidence to support this practice.
- Taking pills does not make up for bad eating habits.
- The fact that Americans spent $28 billion in 2012 on nutritional supplements is more a measure of good marketing than of robust health.

So what is the take-home message from all of this? It's better to spend your time and money improving your diet. This is far more likely to pay off in the long run than popping a pill.

Part of the massive failure of people to pursue exercise is, we believe, the $28 billion supplements industry. How did this industry grow and have such an impact, and how has an industry boomed when there is no compelling evidence to support this practice?

To answer these questions, let's take a brief trip through the supplement business. We have all seen scores of TV ads for supplements. All of them make it appear that the advertised products will have extremely favorable impacts on our lives. Yet we find warnings from the Federal Trade Commission (FTC) produced in cooperation with the Food and Drug Administration (FDA) that make Harvard Medical School's critique seem mild.

These two agencies jointly point out that dietary supplements may seem like harmless health boosters. But while some have proven benefits, many don't. Unlike drugs, dietary supplements aren't evaluated or reviewed by the FDA for either safety or effectiveness. They caution that "even 'natural' supplements can be risky" and that medications you take or the medical conditions you have may make some supplements risky and inappropriate for you in particular. What is worse is that hundreds of supplements have been found to be tainted with drugs and other chemicals. So always talk to your doctor before you take a new supplement, and it is advised that you generally avoid any supplement claiming to be a cure.[24]

You might ask why so many spend their money on this stuff, rather than pursue exercise that is backed up with scientific research. Part of the answer is that exercise is work. And exercise at 75–90 percent intensity exercise is hard work. It is much easier to take a pill that says it will do great things for you without the hard work that delivers great results. And the marketing is very seductive. The following list[25] provided by the FTC lists eight ways to spot supplement fraud. Notice how good they all sound at first blush:

1. Claims that one product does it all and cures a wide variety of health problems.
   - "Proven to treat rheumatism, arthritis, infections, prostate problems, ulcers, cancer, heart trouble, hardening of the arteries and more."

2. Suggestions the product can treat or cure diseases.
   - "Shrinks tumors," "Cures impotency," or "Prevents severe memory loss."

3. Words like scientific breakthrough, miraculous cure, exclusive product, secret ingredient, or ancient remedy.
   - "A revolutionary innovation formulated by using proven principles of natural health-based medical science."

4. Misleading use of scientific-sounding terms.

- "Molecule multiplicity," "glucose metabolism," "thermogenesis," or "insulin receptor sites."

5. Phony references to Nobel Prize–winning technology or science.
   - "Nobel Prize–winning Technology," or "Developed by two-time Nobel Prize winner."

6. Undocumented testimonials by patients or doctors claiming miraculous results.
   - "My husband has Alzheimer's disease. He began eating a teaspoonful of this product each day. And now, in just 22 days, he mowed the grass, cleaned out the garage, weeded the flower beds, and we take our morning walk again."

7. Limited availability and a need to pay in advance.
   - "Hurry. This offer will not last. Send us a check now to reserve your supply."

8. Promises of "no-risk, money-back" guarantees.
   - "If after 30 days you have not lost at least 4 pounds each week, your uncashed check will be returned to you."

There is another reason supplements have soared while exercise languishes. We notice that there is a generation of relatively young, highly successful entrepreneurs and celebrities in the United States who have great lives and want to live forever. They are backing "life-extension" schemes and are enthusiastic about supplements.[26] Search the Internet for "life-extension supplements," and the floodgates will open.

Fred and Steven want to be clear: We both have good health and strength because of what we eat and the exercise we do—not because of growth hormones, testosterone, steroids, vitamins, minerals, or passing-fad substances. We both often have a 30-gram whey protein shake containing the essential amino acids (including leucine and its metabolite HMB) after working out. Steven took vitamin D after heart surgery until a deficiency that appeared in blood tests was addressed. That's it. Fred especially stands apart for having walked the walk long term. At 85 as of August 2017, you will find it difficult to find more than a very few individuals who have lived as long, as well, and strong as Fred.

NO MAGIC PILL CAN REPLACE REAL FOOD OR REAL EXERCISE

We know that intense resistance training increases strength. We also know that such training causes a multitude of extremely complex chemical and other impacts on cells, which make us stronger and healthier. What is happening at the cellular and molecular level is fascinating, and recent research has increasingly been able to peer into this microuniverse. We now see that muscles are much more than simple consumers of nutrients in our bloodstream when they are working. They can also produce a cascade of very sophisticated factors back into our bloodstreams. Skeletal muscles serve as an endocrine gland.[27] They can synthesize and secrete many beneficial growth factors in response to muscle contraction and these factors are necessary for maintenance of whole-body health. Biopsied human skeletal muscle after just one session of high-intensity exercise revealed the appearance of over a thousand unique factors essential in regulating energy and metabolism.

Exercising skeletal muscle triggers many powerful regeneration forces. We asked Dr. Boppart to give us the big picture. She said, "We haven't identified precisely what cell types within the whole muscle tissue contribute to factor release in response to exercise, yet data from our lab and others support a role for stem cells. Stem cells regenerate and repair damaged muscle tissue, yet also secrete small molecules that are important for healing. Immune cells and fibroblasts likely also contribute."

That is the upside, part of the great upward spiral of strength and health that it is possible to trigger by your own behavior. But that is only half the story. The opposite is true, too. Without adequate exercise, you are not just deprived of all of the positive benefits exercise can trigger. No, Dr. Boppart explains, "stem cells and other mononuclear cell types in muscle can begin to secrete factor that is no longer beneficial to muscle or bodily health. Inactivity that occurs with age and disease only serves to compound the problem, eventually leading to extensive loss of muscle mass and strength."

We asked Dr. Boppart to confirm our understanding and asked, "While we don't know all the mechanisms, we do know that exercising the muscles triggers an adaptive response in multiple tissues in the body. If they fall into disuse, not only do they waste from disuse, but they then become a contributor to a decline in whole-body health?"

Her reply was, "Correct."

This important point is counterintuitive. Being sedentary, inactive, is not the same as doing nothing positive for your health; it is a way of hurting yourself, a way to actively damage your health.

Back on the positive side, Dr. Boppart is currently investigating the connection between working muscles and brain health. "If your leg muscles are contracting, for example, and secreting some of these beneficial factors, how do those circulating factors impact the brain?[28] We believe there is specific capacity for muscle-resident stem cells to synthesize and secrete circulating factors during exercise that can promote brain plasticity (the brain's ability to form new neural connections) and this is the focus of some of our current work."

Want an improved memory? Even working out on a treadmill may help.[29]

WHY WON'T A PILL CONTAINING THE SAME GOOD FACTORS WORK?

Dr. Boppart explains, "Single-factor therapies are never effective, and they're not effective because of the complexity of muscle structure and brain circuitry, and the subsequent integration of numerous events necessary for proper function of each tissue type. Exercise can maintain or enhance strength and cognition because multiple systems are activated and synergize with one another, but administration of a single nutrient or molecule will, at best, marginally improve function."

A chemical factor injected always lacks the inherent intelligence and interaction that is part of a living system. It's never the same as a cell that is interacting in real time and providing a far more complicated response to other parts of the body by signaling and communicating, because it's alive and aware, and so the timings, the dosage—everything—is part of an ongoing conversation constantly adjusting the process. The element of an intelligent, living, self-regulating system is lost when we simply inject a dose of a chemical factor or take a pill. We then have shifted to a drug delivery method that will never have the capacity to do this job as well. The process of administering the factor becomes so imprecise and perhaps so ill-timed that more harm than good can easily be done. Dr. Boppart confirms this and adds that "a single-factor therapy will in most cases elicit a negative response rather than have a positive effect."

Want an example? Dr. Boppart says, "Growth hormone would be the best example. Many people now feel that if they inject growth hormone that it will provide the fountain of youth, that it will allow for regeneration of multiple tissues. Unfortunately, when an older adult injects growth hormone, the same changes that occur in a young individual do not occur. Growth hormone may increase the cells in the muscle that can allow for collagen deposition. This means that the overall muscle will grow larger, but the actual muscle tissue that does the work, the myofiber, is not increasing in size, so there's no significant increase in strength—you get a look and no strength—as well as many negative effects, such as edema. Edema is swelling that can occur within that tissue type. I think growth hormone is the perfect example of a single therapy that many perceive as a rejuvenating factor, but this is not the case."

A BIG DIFFERENCE: SUPPLEMENTED VERSUS NATURALLY PRODUCED

How about testosterone? Fred and Steven both exercise their muscles hard and naturally produce plenty of testosterone as a result. Why isn't just injecting testosterone if you have "low T" the same? And if some is good, why isn't more better?

Dr. Boppart warns, "Testosterone therapy has the potential to impact both myofiber growth and strength, even in an aged individual. Unfortunately, though, the negative impact may be increased susceptibility to cancer. Anabolic steroids can elicit a positive impact on cellular division. So, if you have, say, a benign cancer within your body and it's exposed to testosterone, those cells can become malignant. Therefore, we have to be very careful with testosterone. Its use may be beneficial if an individual is clinically deficient in the hormone. It might allow for someone to regain muscle mass and strength without negative impact. But if you have normal levels of testosterone and you're supplementing, that's when the impact can be very dangerous."

If you exercise and your natural testosterone level begins to rise, that is safer, because naturally occurring testosterone is released in the right amount. The body likes to maintain homeostasis, or a balance among your physiological variables (heart rate, blood pressure, concentration of hormones) within a narrow range that allows for a constant internal environment. When any variable is out of balance, the body provides counter-regulatory mechanisms to improve control. The (healthy) body has remarkable capacity to adapt and respond to change. That is part of the system-wide, intelligent, ongoing regulation that a natural system can offer. Its sophistication is not at all replaced by visiting a doctor occasionally.

TOO MUCH IS NOT GOOD

Even vitamins and minerals in high concentration can have negative impact on the body—high doses of vitamin E, for example.[30] Vitamin D is a very hot topic right now. It seems to be essential for metabolic health. However, we now know that if you ingest too much vitamin D, it can increase your risk for heart disease.[31]

Calcium supplementation is strongly promoted. Save your bones! But care is needed there too. A group of urologists that Fred was speaking to recently were discussing new warnings for over-supplementation of calcium because it could trigger heart attacks. Researchers at Johns Hopkins Medicine concluded that taking calcium supplements may harm the heart and vascular system. On the other hand, they found that a diet with lots of calcium-rich foods appeared to be protective.[32]

The bottom line is that concentrations must be within a certain range. If not, otherwise good things may be destructive to the body. Making the effort to get the same nutrients from a healthy diet should be your first choice.

There is yet another problem with supplementation. If we continually take a supplement, we can develop a dependence on the supplement as our natural systems, which would otherwise produce the substance internally in a more intelligently regulated way, tend to shut down because of an artificial abundance of the substance in our system.

We asked Dr. Boppart to provide an example of this process in action. "Supplementation with the antioxidants, such as resveratrol," she said, "is a good example. Aging and disease can provide a challenge to cellular metabolism, or the ability for our cells to convert nutrients into energy. When this occurs, the cell will begin to generate reactive oxygen species (ROS) or oxygen radicals that can destruct tissues, such as muscle. Ingestion of an antioxidant to eliminate ROS would seem to make sense to prevent muscle aging. However, studies have demonstrated that ingestion of large amounts is not only ineffective but may be counterproductive to the beneficial adaptive response associated with exercise. The lesson learned is that the body is 'intelligent,' and it is best not to interfere with a natural stress response. Perhaps consumption of a small amount of red wine, fruits, or vegetables in appropriate amounts may be protective, but supplementation in mega doses may shut down important biological processes."

WHAT WORKS

We asked Dr. Boppart to summarize all of this and reduce it into an overarching health philosophy that could guide good decision-making.

"Proper bodily movement and proper nutrition are the key components of maintenance of systemic health. This information has existed for decades, and everyone is aware. Yet we don't take advantage of this information. One-third of the US population is completely inactive, and another third is insufficiently active to incur any health benefit. This level of inactivity is on par with the rates of individuals who fall into the categories of either overweight or obese. The highest growing rate of inactivity is occurring in school children. Our life has become sedentary, largely due to dependency on computers for news and communication and on the development of other technological advances. The fact that so many people are incurring degenerative-type diseases, such as cardiovascular disease and diabetes, means we must try to reintroduce exercise and proper nutrition into our lifestyle again, and we need to do it immediately.

"As I mentioned previously, exercise releases many beneficial circulating factors that not only impact the muscle itself, the local tissue environment, but also benefit the central nervous system, the liver, the GI tract, and other organ systems. There's no other mechanism that exists that allows you to have such a strong, positive response that is integrative in nature. It simply doesn't exist. We need to incorporate both endurance and strength training into our daily lifestyle. Does that mean that you must go to the gym every day or every other day? No, it is not necessary only to go to the gym. There are so many easy ways to incorporate physical activity into the day. Take the stairs, lift groceries, walk to the park, clean the house, and play outside with the kids. You must decide that this is important to you. You must seek out opportunities for bodily movement. If you're not

"Exercise is the only mechanism that will allow for maintenance of health through the life span. There isn't any other option."

thinking about incorporating exercise in your life, it just won't happen. You will succumb to the sedentary lifestyle. You must determine in your own mind that your health is important and, therefore, that you will make exercise part of your life.

"In all the years I have spent studying physiology and health, I am convinced that exercise is the only mechanism that will allow for maintenance of health through the life span. There isn't any other option."

This is current reality. We have a health-care system that has lost touch with the foundation of health that Dr. Boppart has described well. It has become separated from the exercise and diet it must be built on to be fundamentally sound. It is propped up with money, which may keep us alive, but, minus proper exercise and diet, cannot keep us well and strong as we age. And money to compensate for the bad health effects of inactivity and poor diet choices is drying up.

EVIDENCE OF REVERSING AGING

In the field of molecular biology, gene expression profiling is the measurement of the activity (the expression) of thousands of genes at once, to create a global picture of cellular function. Transcriptional profiling is a procedure that uses arrays on which identified gene sequences are spotted to assay expression in samples of messenger RNA (mRNA).

We asked Dr. Boppart what she found to be the most startling finding so far. This was her reply: "In 2007, a study was published by Simon Melov from the Buck Institute for Age Research (Novato, California) that provided evidence that strength training can reverse the aging process in skeletal muscle. Although previous studies demonstrated improvements in skeletal muscle mass and strength in older adults with training, this study was unique in that it demonstrated a marked impact of exercise on the transcriptional profile of both young and aged skeletal muscle. Overall, the work confirmed the prediction that exercise had an important influence on muscle at the molecular level—and the changes presented were more convincing than reported functional outcomes."

This really does put all the wild claims for all the questionable supplement pills to shame.

"EXERCISE REVERSES AGING IN HUMAN SKELETAL MUSCLE"[33]

This astonishing headline appeared in May 28, 2007. The Buck Institute for Research on Aging faculty in Novato, California, produced a study that, for the first time, physically showed molecular "genetic finger-prints" becoming younger in healthy seniors who did resistance train-ing. In summarizing their results in a release, they emphasized that not only did resistance training make individuals feel better and help them get stronger, it actually also rejuvenated muscle tissue in the already healthy seniors they tested.[34]

This study was the first to directly examine the gene expression profile in their test group. Results first demonstrated a decline in mito-chondrial function in their senior citizen test group. Resistance exer-cise over the period of the study showed "a remarkable reversal" in the genetic fingerprint similar to levels seen in younger adults. Aging studies are typically done on microscopic worms, fruit flies, and mice, where it is permitted to test new chemical agents for effect. It was possible to use humans in this study because there was no potentially dangerous drug being tested.[35]

The faculty expressed great satisfaction in being able to discover and validate something individuals could immediately benefit from that would improve their health and the quality of their lives and reverse aspects of aging.

CASE STUDY: JOSEPH

Between ages 30 and 50, Joseph was a self-described couch potato. "The only exercise I got was when I worked around the house."

He was athletic and fit in his younger years, but as he aged, he simply didn't get around to exercising. He went to the doctor regularly, and initially, there were never any concerns over blood pressure, heart rate, or health-related issues.

But eventually, after decades of taking his eye off the exercise ball, the weight had slowly crept up. Without realizing it, Joseph had gained a lot of weight. He was suddenly 350 pounds—not the fit athlete of his 20s. At age 50, he was uncomfortable, and those medical numbers had also suddenly become alarming. He was told medication was necessary to get his cholesterol and everything else in check.

Joseph was facing serious health consequences for decades of being sedentary.

"It was a gradual progression over time," he said. "You just kind of get used to the lifestyle of being heavy."

But the weight had heavy consequences on his life in addition to his physical health. In one instance, he and his son went to a Notre Dame football game since both are big fans. Walking around, due to the weight, Joseph couldn't keep up. He was tired and sweaty, and ultimately ruined the game for his son because he was so angry at how uncomfortable the weight made him.

And later, a rock-bottom moment: Since he worked in the pharmaceutical industry, Joseph's office had a secure entry system, in which one door opened, a person stepped in, and the back door closed before the next door opened, allowing an employee to enter. But there was a weight requirement—a maximum weight that a person could have to use the door system. Joseph exceeded it. That information was broadcast over a speaker by the security guard one day when Joseph stepped into the first door. Joseph was mortified, and a long line of frustrated workers waiting to get to their desks were held up by Joseph.

Airplanes weren't comfortable for Joseph either, and so he regularly turned down work opportunities that required travel. That impacted his job performance.

Ultimately, Joseph had grown angry, unhappy, and uninspired at work because of his ballooning waistline.

Joseph's brother works for Fred. One day, he was talking to Fred about life at 50. Fred explained that he had turned his entire life around at that age when he tackled strength training hard-core. Fred encouraged Joseph to at least try to do something about his weight and his health.

Joseph listened carefully, taking Fred's words very much to heart.

At first, he started walking, just a bit because that's all he could do. Then he tweaked his diet, gradually eating better.

Joseph is a research scientist, so he is a numbers geek. As he started to see some progress on the scale, he started to track everything in great detail on a spreadsheet. That method of sticking to it worked for him. He weighed himself on the same scale at the same time every day. Then he charted it.

And he made serious progress—the minutes of walking each day turned into an hour at a time, with a desire to keep going for longer. He ate less, and the pounds started slipping away. When the cold weather came, Joseph had built up enough endurance and confidence to get into the gym and eventually started lifting weights.

"I recaptured my youth. For over 20 years, every time I sweat, it was because I was sick or hot," he said. "This was the first time I was actually sweating like I did when I was a kid, because I was doing something, working out and having fun doing it."

Within 8 months, Joseph was down 100 pounds. But the numbers were just half of the win. The reward for his hard work revealed itself in other ways, too.

"Before I lost weight, I was very argumentative. I was angry because my clothes never fit. I couldn't buy the clothes I wanted to buy. I was an outsider. I didn't care about shaving. I didn't care how often I got my hair cut. I didn't care about the clothes that I wore," he said.

Once he felt empowered, he started caring about his appearance and feeling good. And then, Joseph suddenly had unimaginable career prospects when he needed to make a job change.

"I had phone interviews with forty different people, and I ended up having six or seven job interviews, and I got two job offers."

Ultimately, thanks to new confidence, new strength, and weight loss, Joseph landed a big, global job, one that requires he present himself in a professional manner and fly all over the world to conduct business. He was suddenly able and eager to do that.

Today, at 53, he is happy and no longer angry or uncomfortable in his own skin. And he's grateful beyond belief for all that his fitness success has generated.

"I'm the luckiest person in the world," he said.

NOW IT'S YOUR TURN

We are hopeful that our test group's dramatic results, along with all the science and studies with which you've now been armed, have prepped you to dive in and to embrace the StrongPath. If you take only two things away from our study, know this: Results occur quickly, particularly if you are a beginner or have not been exercising seriously for some time. Don't let the gym or your own fear intimidate you. You can do this. To learn more about the StrongPath, visit our website at

Strongpath.com, where you can read additional case studies, download and print our workout logs, watch training videos, and learn about the latest trends in resistance training and nutrition.

> **Results occur quickly, particularly if you are a beginner or have not been exercising seriously for some time. Don't let the gym or your own fear intimidate you.**
>
> **You can do this.**

Notes

Chapter 1

1. National Institute on Aging, National Institutes of Health (NIH), US Department of Health and Human Services, World Health Organization, "Living Longer," *Global Health and Aging* (NIH, 2011), https://www.nia .nih.gov/research/publication/global-health-and-aging/living-longer.

2. Matthew Mezey and Terry Fulmer, "Quality Care for the Frail Elderly," *Nursing Outlook* 46 (1998): 291–292.

3. Paul Jaminet and Shou-Ching Jaminet, "The Rise—and Fall?—of American Health," *Psychology Today* (November 13, 2012), https://www.psychology today.com/blog/perfect-health-diet/201211/the-rise-and-fall-american-health.

4. Amanda Sonnega, "The Future of Human Life Expectancy: Have We Reached the Ceiling or Is the Sky the Limit?" *Research Highlights in the Demography and Economics of Aging* (Population Reference Bureau, 2006), http://www.prb.org/pdf06/NIA_FutureofLifeExpectancy.pdf.

5. National Institute on Aging (NIA), National Institutes of Health, and US Department of Health and Human Services, "Health," *Growing Older in America: The Health and Retirement Study* (NIA, 2007), https://www.nia .nih.gov/health/publication/growing-older-america-health-and-retirement -study/chapter-1-health.

6. Jaminet and Jaminet, 2012.

7.   David Sterman, "Are Pensions Becoming a Thing of the Past?" *Business Insider* (October 30, 2011), http://www.businessinsider.com/pensions -are-a-thing-of-the-past-and-4-other-things-you-need-to-know-to -invest-2011-10.

8.   Elyssa Kirkham, "1 in 3 Americans Has Saved $0 for Retirement," *Money* (March 14, 2016), http://time.com/money/4258451/retirement-savings -survey.

9.   Yagana Shah, "100-Year-Old Athlete Still Does 100 Push-Ups Every Day," *Huffington Post* (June 30, 2015), http://www.huffingtonpost .com/2015/06/30/fred-winter-senior-games-_n_7696848.html.

Chapter 2

1.   Frank W. Booth, Christian K. Roberts, and Matthew J. Laye, "Lack of Exercise Is a Major Cause of Chronic Diseases," *Comprehensive Physiology* 2 (2012): 1143–1211, https://www.ncbi.nlm.nih.gov/pmc/articles /PMC4241367.

2.   Valter Santilli, Andrea Bernetti, Massimiliano Mangone, and Marco Paoloni, "Clinical Definition of Sarcopenia," *Clinical Cases in Mineral and Bone Metabolism* 11 (2014): 177–180, https://www.ncbi.nlm.nih.gov/pmc /articles/PMC4269139.

3.   Josep Maria Argilés, Nefertiti Campos, José M. Lopez-Pedrosa, Ricardo Rueda, and Leocadio Rodriguez-Mañas, "Skeletal Muscle Regulates Metabolism via Interorgan Crosstalk: Roles in Health and Disease," *The Journal of Post-Acute and Long-Term Care Medicine* 17 (2016): 789–796, https://www.ncbi.nlm.nih.gov/pubmed/27324808.

4.   Jane E. Brody, "The Far-Reaching Effects of a Fall," *Well* blog (*New York Times*, 2015), http://well.blogs.nytimes.com/2015/03/09/the-far-reaching -effects-of-a-fall/?_r=0.

5.   Alfonso J. Cruz-Jentoft and John E. Morley (eds.), *Sarcopenia* (Wiley- Blackwell, 2012).

6.   Ibid.

Chapter 3

1. University of Copenhagen, The Faculty of Health and Medical Sciences, "Inactivity reduces people's muscle strength," *ScienceDaily* (June 16, 2015), https://www.sciencedaily.com/releases/2015/06/150626095520.htm.

2. John E. Morley, Angela Marie Abbatecola, Josep M. Argilés, Vickie Baracos, Juergen Bauer, Shalender Bhasin, Tommy Cederholm, Andrew J. Stewart Coats, Steven R. Cummings, William J. Evans, et al, "Sarcopenia with Limited Mobility: An International Consensus," *Journal of the American Medical Directors Association* 12 (2011): 403–409, https://www.ncbi.nlm.nih.gov/pmc/articles/PMC5100674.

3. Li Cao and John E. Morley, "Sarcopenia Is Recognized as an Independent Condition by an International Classification of Disease, Tenth Revision, Clinical Modification (ICD-10-CM) Code," *Journal of the American Medical Directors Association* 17 (2016): 675–677, http://www.jamda.com/article/S1525-8610(16)30181-5/abstract.

4. Alfonso J. Cruz-Jentoft and John E. Morley (eds.), *Sarcopenia* (Wiley-Blackwell, 2012).

5. Ibid.

6. Jonatan R. Ruiz, Xuemei Sui, Felipe Lobelo, James R. Morrow Jr., Allen W. Jackson, Michael Sjöström, and Steven N. Blair, "Association Between Muscular Strength and Mortality in Men: Prospective Cohort Study," *BMJ* 337 (2008): a439, http://www.bmj.com/content/337/bmj.a439.

7. Ibid.

8. Institute on Aging (IOA), "Read How IOA Views Aging in America," IOA website (Institute on Aging, 2017), https://www.ioaging.org/aging-in-america.

9. John E. Morley et al., 2011.

10. Peter Tyson, "Are We Still Evolving?" *NOVA* (PBS 2009), http://www.pbs.org/wgbh/nova/evolution/are-we-still-evolving.html.

11. Daniel Lieberman, *The Story of the Human Body: Evolution, Health, and Disease* (Knopf Doubleday, 2013).

12. Ibid.

13. Frank W. Booth, Manu V. Chakravarthy, and Espen E. Spangenburg,

"Exercise and Gene Expression: Physiological Regulation of the Human Genome Through Physical Activity," *The Journal of Physiology*, 543 (September 1, 2002): 399–411, https://www.ncbi.nlm.nih.gov/pubmed /12205177.

14.   Ibid.

15.   James Gallagher, "Inactivity 'Kills More than Obesity,'" *Health* (BBC News, 2015), http://www.bbc.com/news/health-30812439.

16.   National Institute of Diabetes and Digestive and Kidney Diseases, "Overweight & Obesity Statistics" (NIDDK, 2012), https://www.niddk.nih .gov/health-information/health-statistics/Pages/overweight-obesity -statistics.aspx.

17.   Kelly Wallace, "Teens Spend a 'Mind-Boggling' 9 Hours a Day Using Media, Report Says," CNN.com (November 3, 2015), http://www.cnn .com/2015/11/03/health/teens-tweens-media-screen-use-report.

18.   Thomas E. Ricks, "Military Physical Training: It's a Problem Bigger than Obesity, with No Easy Solutions," *Foreign Policy* (February 18, 2015), http:// foreignpolicy.com/2015/02/18/military-physical-training-its-a-problem -bigger-than-obesity-with-no-easy-solutions.

19.   Ryan Jaslow "Inactivity Tied to 5.2 Million Deaths Worldwide, Similar to Smoking," CBSNews.com (July 18, 2012), http://www.cbsnews.com/news /inactivity-tied-to-53-million-deaths-worldwide-similar-to-smoking.

Chapter 4

1.   Mary Jo Gibson, "Beyond 50.03: A Report to the Nation on Independent Living and Disability: Executive Summary," AARP website (April 2003), http://www.aarp.org/research/health/disabilities/aresearch-import-753.html.

2.   Lynn Feinberg, Susan C. Reinhard, Ari Houser, and Rita Choula, "Valuing the Invaluable: 2011 Update The Growing Contributions and Costs of Family Caregiving," *Insight on the Issues* (AARP Public Policy Institute, July 2011), http://assets.aarp.org/rgcenter/ppi/ltc/i51-caregiving.pdf.

3.   MetLife Mature Market Institute, *Market Survey of Long-Term Care Costs* (MetLife, 2011), https://www.metlife.com/assets/cao/mmi/publications /studies/2011/mmi-market-survey-nursing-home-assisted-living-adult-day -services-costs.pdf.

4.   Genworth, *Genworth 2014 Cost of Care Survey: Executive Summary* (Genworth, 2014), https://www.genworth.com/dam/Americas/US/PDFs /Consumer/corporate/131168-032514-Executive-Summary-nonsecure.pdf.

5.   Richard Barrington, "Survey: Most Americans Underestimate Nursing -Home Costs," MoneyRates.com (June 24, 2014), http://www.money-rates. com/research-center/americans-underestimate-nursing-home-costs.htm.

6.   Katie Thomas, "In Race for Medicare Dollars, Nursing Home Care May Lag," *New York Times* (April 14, 2015), http://www.nytimes.com/2015 /04/15/business/as-nursing-homes-chase-lucrative-patients-quality-of -care-is-said-to-lag.html.

7.   Leah Sottile, "Living Sick and Dying Young in Rich America: Chronic Illness Is the New First-World Problem," *The Atlantic* (December 19, 2013), http://www.theatlantic.com/health/archive/2013/12/living-sick-and-dying -young-in-rich-america/282495.

8.   Ezekial J. Emanuel, "Why I hope to Die at 75: An Argument that Society and Families—and You—Will Be Better Off if Nature Takes Its Course Swiftly and Promptly," *The Atlantic* (October 2014), http://www.theatlantic .com/magazine/archive/2014/10/why-i-hope-to-die-at-75/379329.

9.   Anne Knott and Deirdre Fruh, *The Impact of Chronic Disease on U.S. Health and Prosperity: A Collection of Statistics and Commentary: Almanac of Chronic Disease 2009* (Partnership to Fight Chronic Disease, 2009), http:// www.fightchronicdisease.org/sites/default/files/docs/2009Almanacof ChronicDisease_updated81009.pdf.

10.   Ibid.

11.   Carolyn Y. Johnson, "Health Care Spending Is Projected to Grow Much Faster than the Economy," *Wonkblog* (*The Washington Post*, 2016), https:// www.washingtonpost.com/news/wonk/wp/2016/07/13/health-spending -will-surge-to-encompass-a-huge-chunk-of-the-economy-by-2025/.

12.   Ibid.

13.   National Center for Chronic Disease Prevention and Health Promotion, *The Power of Prevention: Chronic Disease . . . the Public Health Challenge of the 21st Century* (Centers for Disease Control and Prevention, 2009), https://www.cdc.gov/chronicdisease/pdf/2009-power-of-prevention.pdf.

14.   Catherine Le Galès-Camus, Robert Beaglehole, and JoAnne Epping-Jordan (eds.), *Preventing Chronic Diseases: A Vital Investment* (World Health Organization, 2005), http://www.who.int/chp/chronic_disease_report /full_report.pdf.

15.   National Center for Health Statistics, "Exercise or Physical Activity," CDC website (Centers for Disease Control and Prevention, 2017), https://www .cdc.gov/nchs/fastats/exercise.htm.

16.   National Center for Chronic Disease Prevention and Health Promotion, 2009.

17.   Marc Freedman, "How to Make the Most of Longer Lives," *Wall Street Journal* (May 31, 2015), http://www.wsj.com/articles/how-to-make-the -most-of-longer-lives-1432743631.

Chapter 5

1.   Ezekiel J. Emanuel, "Why I hope to Die at 75: An Argument that Society and Families—and You—Will Be Better Off if Nature Takes Its Course Swiftly and Promptly," *The Atlantic* (October 2014), http://www.theatlantic .com/magazine/archive/2014/10/why-i-hope-to-die-at-75/379329.

2.   Ibid.

3.   Ibid.

4.   Teresa E. Seeman, Sharon S. Merkin, Eileen M. Crimmins, and Arun S. Karlamangla, "Disability Trends among Older Americans: National Health and Nutrition Examination Surveys, 1988–1994 and 1999–2004," *American Journal of Public Health* 100 (2010): 100–107, https://www.ncbi.nlm.nih. gov/pubmed/19910350.

5.   Ibid.

6.   Eileen M. Crimmins and Hiram Beltrán-Sánchez, "Mortality and Morbidity Trends: Is There Compression of Morbidity?" *The Journals of Gerontology* 66B (2011): 75–86, https://www.ncbi.nlm.nih.gov/pmc/articles/PMC3001754.

7.   Emanuel, 2014.

8.   Cardiff University, "35 Year Study Finds Exercise Reduces Risk of Dementia," *ScienceDaily* (December 9, 2013), https://www.sciencedaily .com/releases/2013/12/131209181059.htm.

9.   Emanuel, 2014.

10.   Ibid.

11.   Ibid.

12.   Ibid.

13.   Aging in Motion, "Dr. Roger Fielding Gives an Update on Sarcopenia Research," Aging in Motion website, http://aginginmotion.org/dr-roger -fielding-gives-an-update-on-sarcopenia-research.

14.   Patricia M. Barnes and Charlotte A. Schoenborn, "Trends in Adults Receiving a Recommendation for Exercise or Other Physical Activity from a Physician or Other Health Professional," *NCHS Data Brief* 86 (February 2012): 1–8, https://www.ncbi.nlm.nih.gov/pubmed/22617014.

15.   Travis Saunders, "Many Health Impacts of Aging Are Due to Inactivity— Not Getting Old," *MedicalXpress* (June 2, 2015), http://medicalxpress.com /news/2015-06-health-impacts-aging-due-inactivitynot.html.

16.   US Department of Health and Human Services (DHHS), Centers for Disease Control and Prevention, and National Center for Health Statistics, *Summary Health Statistics for U.S. Adults: National Health Interview Survey, 2012,* Vital and Health Statistics series 10 no. 260 (DHHS, 2014), https://www.cdc.gov/nchs/data/series/sr_10/sr10_260.pdf.

17.   Saunders, 2015.

18.   Ibid.

19.   Ibid.

20.   Fay Vincent, "Life as the Ninth Inning Nears," *Wall Street Journal* (February 24, 2016), http://www.wsj.com/articles/life-as-the-ninth-inning -nears-1456359046.

Chapter 6

1.   Christian K. Roberts and R. James Barnard, "Effects of Exercise and Diet on Chronic Disease," *Journal of Applied Physiology* 98 (2005): 3–30, https:// www.ncbi.nlm.nih.gov/pubmed/15591300.

2.   Ibid.

3.   Alfonso J. Cruz-Jentoft and John E. Morley (eds.), *Sarcopenia* (Wiley-Blackwell, 2012).

4.   Ibid.

5.   Ibid.

6.   Alexandra Sifferlin, "Can You Be Fat and Fit—or Thin and Unhealthy?"
        Time (September 5, 2012), http://healthland.time.com/2012/09/05/can-you
        -be-fat-and-fit-or-thin-and-unhealthy.

7.   Daniel Lieberman, *The Story of the Human Body: Evolution, Health, and
        Disease* (Knopf Doubleday, 2013).

8.   Katherine M. Flegal, David F. Williamson, Elsie R. Pamuk, and Harry
        M. Rosenberg, "Estimating Deaths Attributable to Obesity in the United
        States," *American Journal of Public Health* 94 (2004): 1486–1489, https://
        www.ncbi.nlm.nih.gov/pmc/articles/PMC1448478.

9.   Centers for Disease Control and Prevention (CDC), "Adult Obesity Facts,"
        CDC website (September 1, 2016), https://www.cdc.gov/obesity/data/adult
        .html.

10.   Jen Murphy, "Managing Diabetes Risk With Diet and Exercise," *Wall Street
        Journal* (April 4, 2016), http://www.wsj.com/articles/managing-diabetes
        -risk-with-diet-and-exercise-1459783146.

11.   Lieberman, 2013.

12.   Murphy, 2016.

13.   Cleveland Clinic, "Coronary Artery Disease," Cleveland Clinic website
        (March 16, 2017), https://my.clevelandclinic.org/health/articles/coronary
        -artery-disease.

14.   Robert F. Parker, "Physician Advises Knowledge, Exercise, Diet Best
        Approach to Prevent Heart Disease," *Journal of the American College of
        Trial Lawyers* 80 (2016): 31–34.

15.   Jonathan F. Bean and Walter R. Frontera (eds.), *Strength and Power Training:
        A Guide for Adults of All Ages* (Harvard Health Publications, 2015).

16.   Parker, 2016.

17.   New York State Department of Health, "Physical Inactivity and
        Cardiovascular Disease," New York State Department of Health (August
        1999), https://www.health.ny.gov/diseases/chronic/cvd.htm.

18.   Parker, 2016.

19.   Lieberman, 2013.

20. National Institute on Aging (NIA), "Sample Exercises—Endurance," NIA website (January 21, 2016), https://www.nia.nih.gov/health/publication /exercise-physical-activity/sample-exercises-endurance.

21. American Heart Association, "Endurance Exercise (Aerobic)," American Heart Association website (June 6, 2017), http://www.heart.org /HEARTORG/HealthyLiving/PhysicalActivity/FitnessBasics/Endurance -Exercise-Aerobic_UCM_464004_Article.jsp#.WTg_JGjys2w.

22. American Heart Association, "Strength and Resistance Training Exercise," American Heart Association website (March 24, 2015), http://www.heart .org/HEARTORG/HealthyLiving/PhysicalActivity/FitnessBasics/Strength -and-Resistance-Training-Exercise_UCM_462357_Article.jsp#.WGqbu_krI2y.

23. Jonatan R. Ruiz, Xuemei Sui, Felipe Lobelo, Duck-chul Lee, James R. Morrow Jr., Allen W. Jackson, James R. Hébert, Charles E. Matthews, Michael Sjöström, and Steven N. Blair, "Muscular Strength and Adiposity as Predictors of Adulthood Cancer Mortality in Men," *Cancer Epidemiology, Biomarkers, and Prevention* 18 (2009): 1468–1476, http:// cebp.aacrjournals.org/content/18/5/1468.long.

24. Ibid.
    Jason Bardi, "Vigorous Exercise Linked to Gene Activity in Prostate," University of California San Francisco News Center (February 1, 2012), http://www.ucsf.edu/news/2012/02/11438/vigorous-exercise-linked-gene -activity-prostate.

25. National Cancer Institute, "Physical Activity and Cancer," National Cancer Institute (January 27, 2017), http://www.cancer.gov/about-cancer/causes -prevention/risk/obesity/physical-activity-fact-sheet.

26. Ted Schettler, *The Ecology of Breast Cancer: The Promise of Prevention and the Hope for Healing* (CreateSpace 2013).

27. Michelle M. Jung, Graham A. Colditz, Laura C. Collins, Stuart J. Schnitt, James L. Connolly, and Rulla M. Tamimi, "Lifetime Physical Activity and the Incidence of Proliferative Benign Breast Disease," *Cancer Causes and Control* 22 (2011): 1297–1305, https://www.ncbi.nlm.nih.gov/pmc/articles /PMC3363291.

28. National Cancer Institute, 2017.

29.   Adonina Tardon, Won Jin Lee, Miguel Delgado-Rodriguez, Mustafa Dosemeci, Demetrius Albanes, Robert Hoover, and Aaron Blair, "Leisure-Time Physical Activity and Lung Cancer: A Meta-Analysis," *Cancer Causes and Control* 16 (2005): 389–397, https://www.ncbi.nlm.nih.gov/pmc/articles/PMC1255936.

30.   Stacey A. Kenfield, Meir J. Stampfer, Edward Giovannucci, and June M. Chan, "Physical Activity and Survival After Prostate Cancer Diagnosis in the Health Professionals Follow-Up Study," *Journal of Clinical Oncology* 29 (2011): 726–732, http://ascopubs.org/doi/abs/10.1200/jco.2010.31.5226.

31.   Edward L. Giovannucci, Yan Liu, Michael F. Leitzmann, Meir J. Stampfer, and Walter C. Willett, "A Prospective Study of Physical Activity and Incident and Fatal Prostate Cancer," *Archives of Internal Medicine* 165 (2005): 1005–1010, https://www.ncbi.nlm.nih.gov/pubmed/15883238.

32.   Harvard Health Publications, "Abdominal Fat and What to Do about It," Harvard Health Publications website (October 9, 2015), http://www.health.harvard.edu/staying-healthy/abdominal-fat-and-what-to-do-about-it.

33.   Ibid.

34.   Jane E. Brody, "Millions with Leg Pain have Peripheral Artery Disease," *Well* blog (*New York Times*, April 11, 2016), http://well.blogs.nytimes.com/2016/04/11/millions-with-leg-pain-have-peripheral-artery-disease/?_r=0.

35.   Ibid.

36.   International Osteoporosis Foundation (IOF), "Women Over 50 Will Experience Osteoporotic Fractures. As Will Men," *Facts and Statistics* (IOF, 2015), https://www.iofbonehealth.org/facts-statistics.

37.   Kirk L. English and Douglass Paddon-Jones, "Protecting Muscle Mass and Function in Older Adults During Bed Rest," *Current Opinion in Clinical Nutrition and Metabolic Care* 13 (2010): 34–39, https://www.ncbi.nlm.nih.gov/pmc/articles/PMC3276215.

38.   IOF, 2015.

39.   Bean and Frontera, 2015.

40.   Richard A. Friedman, "Can You Get Smarter?" *New York Times* (October 23, 2015), http://www.nytimes.com/2015/10/25/opinion/sunday/can-you-get-smarter.html?_r=0.

41.   Matthew Herper, "Hard Evidence We Can Slow Alzheimer's by Exercising

the Body and the Mind," *Forbes* (July 14, 2014), http://www.forbes.com
/sites/matthewherper/2014/07/14/finally-hard-evidence-that-exercising
-the-body-and-mind-can-slow-dementia/#525a0dfe437d.

42.   Karen Pallarito, "More Evidence that Exercise Is Key to Brain Health,"
Time (July 19, 2011), http://healthland.time.com/2011/07/19/more
-evidence-that-exercise-is-key-to-brain-health.

43.   Laura Donnelly, "One Hour of Exercise a Week 'Can Halve Dementia Risk',"
The Telegraph (July 13, 2014), http://www.telegraph.co.uk/news/health
/news/10964854/One-hour-of-exercise-a-week-can-halve-dementia-risk.html.

44.   Niousha Bolandzadeh, Roger Tam, Todd C. Handy, Lindsay S. Nagamatsu,
Chun Liang Hsu, Jennifer C. Davis, Elizabeth Dao, B. Lynn Beattie, and
Teresa Liu-Ambrose, "Resistance Training and White Matter Lesion
Progression in Older Women: Exploratory Analysis of a 12-Month
Randomized Controlled Trial," *Journal of the American Geriatrics Society*
63 (2015): 2052–2060, https://www.ncbi.nlm.nih.gov/pubmed/26456233.

45.   BBCNews, "Exercise 'Significant Role' in Reducing Risk of Dementia,
Long-Term Study Finds," BBCNews (December 10, 2013), http://www.bbc
.com/news/uk-wales-25303707.

46.   B. M. Brown, J. J. Peiffer, and R. N. Martins, "Multiple Effects of Physical
Activity on Molecular and Cognitive Signs of Brain Aging: Can Exercise
Slow Neurodegeneration and Delay Alzheimer's Disease?" *Molecular
Psychiatry* 18 (2013): 864–874, http://www.nature.com/mp/journal/v18/n8
/full/mp2012162a.html.

47.   Mayo Clinic, "Aerobic Exercise May Reduce the Risk of Dementia
Researchers Say," *ScienceDaily* (September 8, 2011), https://www
.sciencedaily.com/releases/2011/09/110907163919.htm.

48.   Shivani Garg, "Alzheimer Disease and APOE-4," *MedScape* (February 21,
2015), http://emedicine.medscape.com/article/1787482-overview.

49.   Gretchen Reynolds, "Can Exercise Reduce Alzheimer's Risk?" *Well* blog
(*New York Times*, July 2, 2014), http://well.blogs.nytimes.com/2014/07/02
/can-exercise-reduce-alzheimers-risk/?ref=health.

50.   Ibid.

51.   Herper, 2014.

52.   Gretchen Reynolds, "How Exercise Can Strengthen the Brain," *Well* blog

(*New York Times*, September 28, 2011), http://well.blogs.nytimes
.com/2011/09/28/how-exercise-can-strengthen-the-brain/?_r=0.

53.   Ibid.

54.   Ibid.

55.   Ibid.

56.   Lieberman, 2013.

57.   Tetsuo Koyama, John G. McHaffie, Paul J. Laurienti, and Robert C. Coghill, "The Subjective Experience of Pain: Where Expectations become Reality," *Proceedings of the National Academy of Sciences* 102 (2005): 12950–12955, http://www.pnas.org/content/102/36/12950.full.

58.   W. Timothy Gallwey, *The Inner Game of Golf* (Random House, 2009).

Chapter 7

1.   Erin (Mack) McKelvey, "New Year's Resolutions Won't Make You More Successful," *Fortune* (January 6, 2016), http://fortune.com/2016/01/06/new-years-resolutions-successful.

2.   Jonah Lehrer, "Blame It on the Brain," *The Wall Street Journal* (December 26, 2009), http://www.wsj.com/articles/SB10001424052748703478704574612052322122442.

3.   Carol A. Seger and Brian J. Spiering, "A Critical Review of Habit Learning and the Basal Ganglia." *Frontiers in Systems Neuroscience* 5 (2011): 66, http://www.ncbi.nlm.nih.gov/pmc/articles/PMC3163829.

4.   Becca R. Levy, Suzanne R. Kunkel, and Stanislav V. Kasl, "Longevity Increased by Positive Self-Perceptions of Aging," *Journal of Personality and Social Psychology* 83 (2002): 261–270, http://www.apa.org/pubs/journals/releases/psp-832261.pdf.

5.   Becca R. Levy, Martin D. Slade, Terrence E. Murphy, and Thomas M. Gill, "Association between Positive Age Stereotypes and Recovery from Disability in Older Persons," *JAMA* 308 (2012): 1972–1973, http://jamanetwork.com/journals/jama/fullarticle/1392557.

6.   Daniel Duane, "How the Other Half Lifts: What Your Workout Says about Your Social Class," *Pacific Standard* (July 23, 2014), https://psmag.com

/how-the-other-half-lifts-what-your-workout-says-about-your-social-class
-f04d1b70c507#.oqieres81.

7.   Michael R. Esco, *Resistance Training for Health and Fitness* (American
College of Sports Medicine, 2013), https://www.acsm.org/docs/brochures
/resistance-training.pdf.

Chapter 8

1.   Melinda Wenner, "Smile! It Could Make You Happier," *Scientific American*
(September 1, 2009), https://www.scientificamerican.com/article/smile-it
-could-make-you-happier.

2.   Jonathan F. Bean and Walter R. Frontera (eds.), *Strength and Power Training:
A Guide for Adults of All Ages* (Harvard Health Publications, 2015).

3.   Melinda Beck, "Conquering Fear," *Wall Street Journal* (January 2, 2011),
http://online.wsj.com/news/articles/SB1000142405274870411150457605982
3679423598.

4.   Melanie Gibson, "Discipline of the Body and Mind: Using Martial Arts
Forms as Moving Meditation," BookMartialArts.com (July 19, 2016),
https://www.bookmartialarts.com/news/discipline-of-the-body-and-mind
-using-martial-arts-forms-as-moving-meditation.

5.   Victoria Tilney McDonough, "Beyond Chanting 'Om': The Power Behind
Mindfulness-Based Mind Fitness Training for Soldiers," brainlinemilitary.org
(2014), http://www.brainlinemilitary.org/content/2014/08/beyond-chanting
-om-the-power-behind-mindfulness-based-mind-fitness-training-for.html.

6.   Center for Security Studies, " Using Mind Fitness," Georgetown University
School of Foreign Service (January 29, 2013), https://css.georgetown.edu
/story/1242694602343.

7.   Georgia Paige, "Balanced Fitness, Tougher Brain," *Oxygen* (October 21,
2014), http://www.oxygenmag.com/article/balanced-fitness-tougher
-brain-8644.

8.   Center for Security Studies, 2013.

9.   Matthew Chan, "Growing Stronger—Strength Training for Older Adults
(CDC)," Matthew Chan training log blog (February 24, 2011), http://
chanmatthewchan.com/traininglog/growing-stronger-strength-training
-for-older-adults-cdc.

Chapter 9

1. Stuart Oskamp and P. Wesley Schultz, *Attitudes and Opinions* (Psychology Press, 3rd ed., 2004): 71.

2. Gemma Calvert, "Everything You Need to Know about Implicit Reaction Time (IRTs)," Gemma's Blog (2015), http://gemmacalvert.com/everything -you-need-to-know-about-implicit-reaction-time.

3. Herman Melville, *Moby Dick: Or, The White Whale* (St. Botolph Society, 1892): 267.

4. William James, "Habit," chapter 4 in *The Principles of Psychology* (Holt 1890), http://psychclassics.yorku.ca/James/Principles/prin4.htm.

5. Phillippa Lally, Cornelia H. M. van Jaarsveld, Henry W. W. Potts, and Jane Wardle, "How Are Habits Formed: Modelling Habit Formation in the Real World," *European Journal of Social Psychology* 40 (2010): 998–1009, http:// onlinelibrary.wiley.com/doi/10.1002/ejsp.674/abstract.

6. Jonah Lehrer, "Blame It on the Brain," *Wall Street Journal* (December 26, 2009), http://online.wsj.com/article/SB1000142405274870347870457461205 2322122442.html#printMode.

7. Gina Kolata, "Don't Starve a Cold of Exercise," *New York Times* (December 24, 2008), http://www.nytimes.com/2008/12/25/health/nutrition/25best.html.

8. Benjamin Libet, *Mind Time: The Temporal Factor in Consciousness* (Harvard University Press, 2005): 93.

9. Michael J. Mahoney, *Human Change Processes: The Scientific Foundations of Psychotherapy* (Basic Books, 1991): 427–435.

Chapter 10

1. Robert R. Wolfe, "The Underappreciated Role of Muscle in Health and Disease," *The American Journal of Clinical Nutrition* 84 (2017): 475–482, http://ajcn.nutrition.org/content/84/3/475.full.

2. Enrique Rivero, "Older Adults: Build Muscle and You'll Live Longer," *UCLA Newsroom* (March 13, 2014), http://newsroom.ucla.edu/portal/ucla /older-adults-build-muscle-and-271651.aspx.

3. Martin Nilsson, Joel Eriksson, Berit Larsson, Anders Odén, Helena Johansson, and Mattias Lorentzon, "Fall Risk Assessment Predicts Fall-Related Injury, Hip Fracture, and Head Injury in Older Adults," *Journal of*

the American Geriatrics Society 64 (2016): 2242–2250, https://www.ncbi .nlm.nih.gov/pubmed/27689675.

4. Jonathan F. Bean and Walter R. Frontera (eds.), *Strength and Power Training: A Guide for Adults of All Ages* (Harvard Health Publications, 2015).

5. Centers for Disease Control and Prevention (CDC), "Physical Activity and Health: A Report of the Surgeon General: Adults," CDC website (November 17, 1999), http://www.cdc.gov/nccdphp/sgr/adults.htm.

6. Ibid.

7. Centers for Disease Control and Prevention (CDC), "Physical Activity and Health: A Report of the Surgeon General: Adolescents and Young Adults," *Physical Activity and Health: A Report of the Surgeon General,* CDC website (November 17, 1999), https://www.cdc.gov/nccdphp/sgr/adoles.htm.

8. Ibid.

9. Stephen Seiler, "Basic Skeletal Muscle Physiology: The Motor Unit," *Exercise Physiology* (2017), http://www.time-to-run.com/physiology /skeletal-muscle/motor.htm.

10. Bean and Frontera, 2015.

Chapter 11

1. Harvard Health Publications, "Do You Need to See a Doctor before Starting Your Exercise Program?" Harvard Health Publications website (2017), http://www.health.harvard.edu/healthbeat/do-you-need-to-see-a -doctor-before-starting-your-exercise-program.

2. Seek out board-certified trainers who may specialize in your age group, athletic level, or injury.

3. Jack M. Guralnik, *Assessing Physical Performance in the Older Patient* (National Institute on Aging, 2013), https://www.irp.nia.nih.gov/branches /leps/sppb.

4. Stephanie Studenski, Subashan Perera, Dennis Wallace, Julie M. Chandler, Pamela W. Duncan, Earl Rooney, Michael Fox, and Jack M. Guralnik, "Physical Performance Measures in the Clinical Setting," *Journal of the American Geriatrics Society* 51 (2003): 314–322, https://www.ncbi.nlm.nih .gov/pubmed/12588574.

5. Ibid.

6.   Guralnik, 2013.

7.   Ibid.

8.   Functional Movement System website, http://www.functionalmovement
      .com.

Chapter 12

1.   J. Kruger, S. Carlson, and H. Kohl III, "Trends in Strength Training—
      United States, 1998–2004," *Morbidity and Mortality Weekly Report* 55
      (2006): 769–772, http://www.cdc.gov/mmwr/preview/mmwrhtml
      /mm5528a1.htm.

2.   GlobalNewswire, "SilverSneakers celebrates 25 Years of Changing Lives"
      Nasdaq website (April 19, 2017), http://www.nasdaq.com/press-release
      /silversneakers-celebrates-25-years-of-changing-lives-20170419-00798.
      NewsOK, "The Cost of Getting Exercise," NewsOK website (November 8,
      2016), http://newsok.com/article/5526056.

Chapter 13

1.   Mayo Clinic, "Overexerting Yourself," Mayo Clinic website (May 19, 2017),
      http://www.mayoclinic.org/healthy-lifestyle/fitness/in-depth/exercise
      -intensity/art-20046887?pg=2.

2.   Andrew C. Fry, "The Role of Resistance Exercise Intensity on Muscle Fibre
      Adaptations," *Sports Medicine* 34 (2004): 663–679, https://www.ncbi.nlm
      .nih.gov/pubmed/15335243.

3.   Tony Bonvechio, "Master the Hip Hinge, Exercise's Most Important
      Motion," Stack.com (March 26, 2014), http://www.stack.com/expert/tony
      -bonvechio?page=4.

Chapter 14

1.   Bryan Miller, "How Crash Diets Harm Your Health," CNN Health (April 20,
      2010), http://www.cnn.com/2010/HEALTH/04/20/crash.diets.harm.health.

2.   Rory Heath, "Does Strength Training Build Stronger Bones?" Strength and
      Conditioning Research.com, https://www.strengthandconditioningresearch
      .com/perspectives/strength-training-stronger-bones.

3.   Kathleen M. Zelman, "7 Things Never to Do to Lose Weight," WebMD (April 5, 2014), http://www.webmd.com/diet/obesity/features/lose-weight-dangers.

4.   Gina Kolata, "After 'The Biggest Loser,' Their Bodies Fought to Regain Weight," *New York Times* (May 2, 2016), http://www.nytimes.com/2016 /05/02/health/biggest-loser-weight-loss.html.

5.   Andres Ayesta, "The Best Protein Article Ever!" Vive Nutrition website (November 24, 2015), http://www.vive-nutrition.com/#!The-best-protein -article-ever/hxicq/5654d3fa0cf2b6a6e9316d24.

6.   Douglas Paddon-Jones, Wayne W Campbell, Paul F Jacques, Stephen B Kritchevsky, Lynn L Moore, Nancy R Rodriguez, and Luc JC van Loon, "Protein and Healthy Aging," *American Journal of Clinical Nutrition* 101 (2015): 13395–13455, http://ajcn.nutrition.org/content/early/2015/04/29 /ajcn.114.084061.full.pdf.

7.   Douglas Paddon-Jones and Blake B. Rasmussen, "Dietary Protein Recommendations and the Prevention of Sarcopenia," *Current Opinion in Clinical Nutrition and Metabolic Care* 12 (2009): 86–90, https://www.ncbi .nlm.nih.gov/pubmed/19057193.

8.   University of Texas Medical Branch (UTMB), "Moderate Amounts of Protein per Meal Found Best for Building Muscle," UTMB Health (October 26, 2009), https://www.utmb.edu/newsroom/article5451.aspx.

9.   Paddon-Jones et al., 2015.

10.   Ibid.

11.   Il-Young Kim, Scott Schutzler, Amy Schrader, Horace Spencer, Patrick Kortebein, Nicolaas E. P. Deutz, Robert R. Wolfe, and Arny A. Ferrando, "Quantity of Dietary Protein Intake, but Not Pattern of Intake, Affects Net Protein Balance Primarily through Differences in Protein Synthesis in Older Adults," *American Journal of Physiology—Endocrinology and Metabolism* 308 (2014): E21–E28, http://ajpendo.physiology.org/content/308/1/E21.

12.   Ibid.

13.   Elfego Galvan, Emily Arentson-Lantz, Séverine Lamon, and Douglas Paddon-Jones, "Protecting Skeletal Muscle with Protein and Amino Acid During Periods of Disuse," *Nutrients* 8 (2016): 404. https://www.ncbi.nlm .nih.gov/pmc/articles/PMC4963880.

14. George A. Bray, Steven R. Smith, Lilian de Jonge, Hui Xie, Jennifer Rood, Corby K. Martin, Marlene Most, Courtney Brock, Susan Mancuso, and Leanne M. Redman, "Effect of Dietary Protein Content on Weight Gain, Energy Expenditure, and Body Composition During Overeating," *JAMA* 307 (2012): 47–55, https://www.ncbi.nlm.nih.gov/pmc/articles/PMC3777747.

15. Ibid.

16. Shane Bilsborough and Neil J. Mann, "A Review of Issues of Dietary Protein Intake in Humans," *International Journal of Sport Nutrition and Exercise Metabolism* 16 (2006): 129–152, https://www.ncbi.nlm.nih.gov /pubmed/16779921.

17. Ibid.

18. Tiffany O'Callaghan, "Cured, Smoked Meat Linked with Heart Disease Risk," *Time* (May 17, 2010), http://healthland.time.com/2010/05/17/cured -smoked-meat-linked-with-heart-disease-risk.

19. Harvard T. H. Chan School of Public Health, "Protein," *The Nutrition Source* (Harvard, 2017), https://www.hsph.harvard.edu/nutritionsource/what -should-you-eat/protein.

20. Paddon-Jones et al., 2015.

21. Ibid.

22. David A. Raichlen and Gene E. Alexander, "Exercise, APOE Genotype, and the Evolution of the Human Lifespan," *Trends in Neurosciences* 37 (2014): 247–255, https://www.ncbi.nlm.nih.gov/pmc/articles/PMC4066890.

23. Dariush Mozaffarian (ed.), *Making Sense of Vitamins and Minerals: Choosing the Foods and Nutrients You Need to Stay Healthy* (Harvard Medical School, 2015).

24. Federal Trade Commission, "Dietary Supplements," Federal Trade Commission website (November 2011), https://www.consumer.ftc.gov /articles/0261-dietary-supplements.

25. Ibid.

26. Yehui Duan, Fengna Li, Yinghui Li, Yulong Tang, Xiangfeng Kong, Zemeng Feng, Tracy G. Anthony, Malcolm Watford, Yongqing Hou, Guoyao Wu, and Yulong Yin, "The Role of Leucine and its Metabolites in

Protein and Energy Metabolism," *Amino Acids* 48 (2016): 41–51, https://
www.ncbi.nlm.nih.gov/pubmed/26255285.

27.   Bente K. Pedersen and Mark A. Febbraio, "Muscle as an Endocrine Organ:
Focus on Muscle-Derived Interleukin-6," *Physiological Review* 88 (2008):
1379–1406, https://www.ncbi.nlm.nih.gov/pubmed/18923185.

28.   Heidi Godman, "Regular Exercise Changes the Brain to Improve Memory,
Thinking Skills," Harvard Health Publications website (November 9, 2016),
http://www.health.harvard.edu/blog/regular-exercise-changes-brain
-improve-memory-thinking-skills-201404097110.

29.   Hyo Youl Moon, Andreas Becke, David Berron, Benjamin Becker, Nirnath
Sah, Galit Benoni, Emma Janke, Susan T. Lubejko, Nigel H. Greig, Julie
A. Mattison, Emrah Duzel, and Henriette van Praag, "Running-Induced
Systemic Cathepsin B Secretion Is Associated with Memory Function,"
Cell Metabolism 24 (2016): 332–340, https://www.ncbi.nlm.nih.gov
/pubmed/27345423.

30.   National Institutes of Health (NIH), Office of Dietary Supplements,
"Vitamin E Fact Sheet for Consumers," NIH website (May 9, 2016), https://
ods.od.nih.gov/factsheets/VitaminE-Consumer/#h8.

31.   Katherine Zeratsky, "What Is Vitamin D Toxicity, and Should I Worry
about It since I Take Supplements?" Mayo Clinic website (February 5,
2015), http://www.mayoclinic.org/healthy-lifestyle/nutrition-and-healthy
-eating/expert-answers/vitamin-d-toxicity/faq-20058108.

32.   Johns Hopkins Medicine, "Calcium Supplements May Damage the Heart,"
Johns Hopkins Medicine website (October 11, 2016), http://www.hopkins
medicine.org/news/media/releases/calcium_supplements_may_damage
_the_heart.

33.   Buck Institute for Research on Aging, "Exercise Reverses Aging in Human
Skeletal Muscle," Buck Institute website (May 28, 2007), http://www.buck
institute.org/buck-news/exercise-reverses-aging-human-skeletal-muscle.

34.   Ibid.

35.   Ibid.

Index

About the Authors

FRED BARTLIT

Fred is a West Point graduate, a US Army troop commander, and a US Army Ranger. He was first in his class in law school and holds the top academic record in the 120-year history of the University of Illinois College of Law. Fred is the subject of many books and publications, including *America's Top Trial Lawyers: Who They Are and Why They Win*, *ABA Journal*, and *The National Law*.

Fred has tried over one hundred major cases in twenty-four states, the Virgin Islands, and Scotland. In 2001, he was selected by President Bush to represent him in the presidential election "hanging chad" trial. And in 2010, he was selected by President Obama to be the president's chief counsel for the National Commission on the BP *Deepwater Horizon* Gulf of Mexico oil spill.

Fred has been on the StrongPath for 34 years. *Choosing the StrongPath* is his first book. To reach Fred or to learn more about the StrongPath, visit Strongpath.com.

STEVEN DROULLARD

Steven is a National Academy of Broadcasting graduate and was a news reporter in Washington, DC, during the Watergate era at WPIK/WXRA. Steven was the director of COLL, a mindfulness-based commune during the mid-1970s. He also is a graduate of the Gemological Institute of America and became the CEO of Intergem, Inc. Steven got his master's in consciousness studies from the University of Philosophical Research in Los Angeles, California, where he is now a faculty member. He is also chief business advisor to William R. Hearst II and has been a consultant to the board of directors of the New York Diamond Dealers Club.

Steven was among the first to identify the newly emerging attention economy and worked closely with Sylvain Ringer, a director of the New York Diamond Dealers Club, on its practical implications for the diamond industry. In 2005, Steven introduced the dynamics and mechanics of the developing attention economy to the Diamond Industry Steering Committee.

Steven authored *The Power of Attention* in support of his course in attention mechanics in 2005. Steven and Fred began working together in 2003. Fred taught Steven the powerful impact that serious strength training has on physical and mental fitness. Steven has been on the StrongPath for 12 years. *Choosing the StrongPath* is his second book.

MARNI BOPPART, SCD

Marni Boppart obtained her bachelor degree in molecular, cellular, and developmental biology from the University of New Hampshire in Durham. She obtained her master's degree in cell biology from Creighton University in Omaha, Nebraska, while serving as an officer and aerospace physiologist in the US Air Force. She received her ScD in applied anatomy and physiology from Boston University and completed research for her degree at the Joslin Diabetes Center, Harvard Medical School. Her postdoctoral work was completed in the Department of Cell and Developmental Biology at the University of Illinois, Urbana–Champaign. She is an associate professor in the Department of Kinesiology and Community Health and is full-time faculty at the Beckman Institute for Advanced Science and Technology at the University of Illinois, Urbana–Champaign, where she heads the Molecular Muscle Physiology Laboratory.

Her research interests include cellular biomechanics, cell signaling, and the role of extracellular matrix proteins in the protection of skeletal muscle from injury, disease, and aging.